# Essentials of Diabetes Medicine

LESLIE BAHN KAWA

AuthorHouse™ UK
1663 Liberty Drive
Bloomington, IN 47403  USA
www.authorhouse.co.uk
UK TFN: 0800 0148641 (Toll Free inside the UK)
UK Local: 02036 956322 (+44 20 3695 6322 from outside the UK)

Because of the dynamic nature of the Internet, any web addresses or links contained in this book may have changed since publication and may no longer be valid. The views expressed in this work are solely those of the author and do not necessarily reflect the views of the publisher, and the publisher hereby disclaims any responsibility for them.

Any people depicted in stock imagery provided by Getty Images are models, and such images are being used for illustrative purposes only.
Certain stock imagery © Getty Images.

This book is printed on acid-free paper.

ISBN: 978-1-6655-9764-7 (sc)
ISBN: 978-1-6655-9765-4 (e)

Print information available on the last page.

Published by AuthorHouse 05/22/2023

authorHOUSE®

# Essentials of Diabetes Medicine

# Dedication

*To my wife, Maggie, and our four children,
McClee, Tamara, Zarrah, and Briah*

# Acknowledgement

This book has been a project designed after the completion of the Postgraduate Diploma in Diabetes Medicine from the University of Leicester, United Kingdom, accredited by the International Diabetes Federation. The structure of the book has been designed to reflect the discussions made by the students and the tutors at the time and I would like to acknowledge their contributions.

I also would like to acknowledge the Author House Editorial and the Support teams for the edition, designing and the support provided throughout the process of the publication. Finally, this project wouldn't have been successful without the support of my family.

# Disclaimer

The author has endeavoured to ensure that this book was written with all up-to-date information. However, with increasing evidence and subtle changes in practice, the readership might find some information obsolete. It is, therefore, recommended that the readership seek further information on the subject matter. The author does not accept any culpability for an incorrect clinical decision based on any aspects of this book.

# Essentials of Diabetes Medicine

**Leslie Bahn Kawa *MSc, MRCP UK, FRCP Edin.***
Consultant Physician Acute & General Internal Medicine
East Sussex NHS Trust
United Kingdom

# Preface

Diabetes is a global epidemic affecting all levels of societies and is expected to rise in the coming decades. The rising incidences of diabetes, especially the type 2 diabetes, continue unabated as the population increases and turn to the 'westernised lifestyle' and away from the traditional lifestyle. It is a disease with high financial burden, costing individuals and the healthcare systems throughout the world, billions of dollars. The human costs—loss of lives and poor quality of life are immeasurable.

Recent medical advances made in understanding the pathophysiology, treatment, and optimal management strategies have transformed diabetes from a fatal disease into a chronic illness that is essentially self-manageable by patients. Patient's education on lifestyle, exercise prescriptions, and management of diabetes with the new armaments have shown to improve outcomes.

Management of diabetes in the developed world is not as easy as it may seem; physicians and patients' psychological inertias, non-compliance, and complex management of complications are some barriers that affect the disease outcome.

Management of diabetes in the developing world where two-thirds of the diabetes population live is extremely difficult. Lack of appropriate healthcare institutions, trained professionals, and resources poses greater challenges in managing this epidemic. Addressing these issues in a holistic manner will lead to proper control and management of the epidemic.

Diabetes training and education for all healthcare workers is one of the cornerstones of addressing this epidemic. For this reason, this book has been written purposely to impart to the healthcare professionals the necessary knowledge and tools to manage their diabetes patients appropriately and optimally. It is also expected to be a resourceful material for those embarking in studies related to diabetes.

The concepts and management strategies written in this book, if understood and applied at the bedside by any healthcare professionals, then the management of patients with diabetes can be an enjoyable journey for both the patients and their health careers. And I would have achieved my objective in writing *Essentials of Diabetes Medicine*.

# List of Abbreviations

**ABI**. ankle-brachial index
**ACCORD**. Action to Control Cardiovascular Risks in Diabetes Trial
**ACE-I**. angiotensin-converting-enzyme inhibitors
**ACOG**. American College of Obstetrics and Gynaecology
**ACSM**. American College of Sports Medicine
**ADA**. American Diabetes Association
**AGEs**. advanced glycation end products
**AHA**. American Heart Association
**ARB**. angiotensin receptor blockers
**ATP**. adenosine triphosphate
**ATP III**. Adult Treatment Panel III
**BG**. blood glucose
**BMI**. body mass index
**CAD**. coronary artery disease
**CABG**. coronary artery bypass graft
**CBG**. capillary blood glucose
**CCB**. calcium channel blockers
**CCM**. chronic care model
**CIIP**. continuous insulin infusion pump
**CRF**. chronic renal failure
**CSIIP**. continuous subcutaneous insulin pump
**CVE**. cardiovascular events
**CVD**. cardiovascular disease
**DAFNE**. dose adjustment for normal eating
**DCCT**. Diabetes Control and Complication Trial
**DESMOND**. diabetes education and self-management for newly diagnosed diabetes
**DKA**. diabetes ketoacidosis
**DPP**. American Diabetes Prevention Program
**DPP4**. diethyl peptide peptidase 4
**DR**. diabetic retinopathy
**DPS**. Finnish Diabetes Prevention Study
**EASD**. European Association of Study of Diabetes
**ESRF**. End-stage renal failure
**FFA**. free fatty acids
**FPG**. fasting plasma glucose
**FRII**. fixed rate insulin infusion
**GADA**. glutamic acid decarboxylase autoantibody
**GDM**. gestational diabetes mellitus
**GFR**. glomerular filtration rate
**GIP**. glucose-dependent insulinotrophic peptide

**GLP-1**. Glucagon-like peptide 1

**GLP-1RA**. Glucagon-like peptide 1 receptor antagonist

**HAF**. hypoglycaemic autonomic failure

**HBA1c**. Glycated Hemoglobin A1c

**HBM**. health belief model

**HCP**. healthcare provider

**HHS**. hyperosmolar hyperglycaemic state

**IAA**. insulin autoantibodies

**IA-2**. islet tyrosine phosphate 2

**ICA**. islet cell autoantibodies

**IDF**. International Diabetes Federation

**IDPP**. Indian Diabetes Prevention Program

**IFG**. impaired fasting glucose

**IGT**. impaired glucose tolerance

**IHSG**. International Hypoglycaemic Study Group

**KPD**. ketosis prone diabetes

**LADA**. latent autoimmune disease in adult

**LDL-C**. low density lipoprotein cholesterol

**MDT**. multidisciplinary team

**MODY**. maturity-onset diabetes of the young

**MRI**. magnetic resonance imaging

**NATA**. National Athletic Trainer's Association

**NCEP III**. National Cholesterol Evaluation Program

**NICE**. National Institute of Clinical Excellence

**OGTT**. oral glucose tolerance test

**PCI**. percutaneous coronary intervention

**PNG**. Papua New Guinea

**PNG IMR**. PNG Institute of Medical Research

**PPG**. postprandial glucose

**PVD**. peripheral vascular disease

**RRT**. renal replacement therapy

**SAT**. subcutaneous adipose tissue

**SBGM**. serum blood glucose monitoring

**SCT**. social cognitive theory

**SGLT2**. sodium glucose transporters 2

**STOP NIDDM**. Study To Prevent NIDDM (STOP-NIDDM) Trial

**T2DM**. Type 2 diabetes mellitus

**T1DM**. Type 1 diabetes mellitus

**UKPDS**. United Kingdom Prospective Diabetes Study

**VRII**. variable rate insulin infusion

**WHO**. World Health Organization

**XENDOS**. Xenical in the Prevention of Diabetes in Obese Subjects (XENDOS) study

# Contents

# CHAPTER 1

# Epidemiology of Diabetes Mellitus

Walk for the cure? Wouldn't it be faster if we ran?
**Unknown Author**

## Global Diabetes Epidemiology

Diabetes is a global epidemic that continues to affect millions of people worldwide.[1] There are approximately 285 million people with diabetes worldwide, and that number is expected to reach 438 million by the year 2030.[2] According to the World Health Organisation (WHO) and the International Diabetes Federation (IDF), 3.2 million deaths every year are related to diabetes, and more than 50% of the epidemic is in the developing countries (**Fig.1.1**). This is because of the rising incidences and prevalence of diabetes in China and the Indian subcontinent.

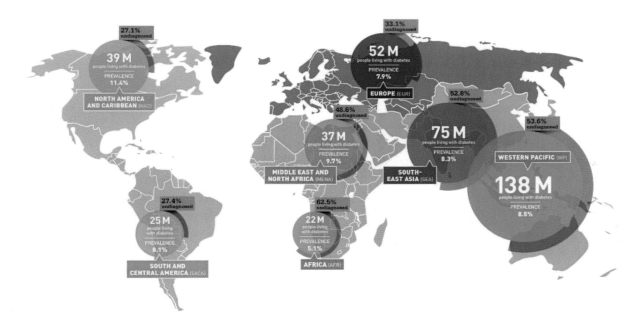

Figure 1.1 Global incidence and prevalence of diabetes. Reproduced with permission from International Diabetes Federation. IDF Diabetes Atlas, 10th edition, Brussels, Belgium: International Diabetes Federation, 2021. http://www.diabetesatlas.org

## Regional Diabetes Epidemiology

The Pacific Region is noted as one of the regions with the highest prevalence of diabetes. According to a WHO bulletin, diabetes prevalence ranges between 14 and 44% in the region. Even Pacific Islanders living abroad have been shown to have high incidences of diabetes. [3]

## National Diabetes Epidemiology

Papua New Guinea (PNG) has a predominantly type 2 diabetes mellitus (T2DM) population with a significant number of undiagnosed cases and impaired fasting glucose (IFG) among the population.

A WHO survey in 2004 showed an incidence of IFG at 14.9% among working-class population in Port Moresby.[4] Recent community survey by the PNG's Medical Research Institute (IMR) showed a 19.7% increase in IFG among both the urban and rural communities.[5] This shows that the incidence and prevalence are rising and affecting all levels of societies and is expected to rise in the coming decades as people adopt a westernised lifestyle—lack of exercise and increased intake of foods rich in sugar and saturated fatty acids. The Port Moresby General Hospital data shows that diabetes-related morbidity and mortality is the highest among all the non-communicable diseases at 17% (unpublished audit).[6]

## Mechanism of Diabetes Epidemic

Although the mechanism behind the cause of diabetes through the adoption of the westernised diet and lack of exercise is not known, it has generally been shown that changing this lifestyle behaviour could potentially prevent diabetes among the high-risk groups. [7-8] It has also been shown to control overt diabetes and even remit diabetes leading to cessation of drug therapy. [9]

## Potential Therapeutic Approach to Curbing the Diabetes Epidemic

Dieting, exercise, and pharmacotherapies remain the three pillars of diabetes management. Randomised clinical trials show that diabetes is preventable among the high-risk groups of different populations in different geographies with dieting, exercise, and pharmacotherapy.

A low-carbohydrate diet with minimum exercise (brisk walking) of 150 minutes every week is recommended for reducing diabetes. Supervised aerobic exercises lead to increased insulin sensitivity that lasts for twenty-four to seventy-two hours, whilst the anaerobic strength exercises improve other cardiovascular risk factors such as the reduction of blood pressure (by 5 mmHg systolic and 2.5 mmHg diastolic pressures), improvement in lipid profile, and muscle toning.

In addition, metformin has been shown to prevent diabetes in the high-risk population, and the American Diabetes Association (ADA) has recommended metformin as the only drug to be used as prophylaxis among the high-risk group since 2006.

## Key Messages:

- **Diabetes is a global epidemic with its epicentre shifted to the Asia-Pacific Region.**
- **The adoption of a westernised lifestyle and improved lifespan have increased diabetes prevalence.**
- **Lifestyle modifications and pharmacoprophylaxis will lead to reduction in the epidemic.**

## References:

1	International Diabetes Federation, 'IDF Diabetes Atlas', Epidemiology and Morbidity. https://www.idf.org/.

2	World Health Organisation and IDF, 'Diabetes Action Now', An Initiative of the WHO and IDF. https://www.who.int/diabetes/actionnow/.

3	Pacific islanders pay heavy price for abandoning traditional diet. (2010). *Bulletin of the World Health Organization, 88(7)*, 484–485. https://doi.org/10.2471/BLT.10.010710

4	Papua New Guinea National Department of Health. *Diabetes Survey* (unpublished). Waigani, Government Printers. 2009.

5	Pulford J, Rarau P, Vengiau G, Gouda H, Phuanukoonnon S & the Scientific Advisory Board. Non-Communicable Diseases and Associated Risk Factors in the Hiri, Asaro and Karkar Integrated Health and Demographic Surveillance Sites (2015). Papua New Guinea Institute of Medical Research, Goroka. https://www.pngimr.org.pg/wp-content/uploads/2019/05 /Report-on-Non-Communicable-diseases-associated-risk-factors-in-the-Hiri-Karkar-and-Asaro-integrated-health-and-demographic-surveillance-sites.pdf.

6	*Annual Audit Report* (2011). Division of Internal Medicine, Port Moresby General Hospital.

7	G. Sartor, B. Schersten, S. Carlstrom, et al., 'Ten-Year Follow-Up of Subjects with Impaired Glucose Tolerance. Prevention of Diabetes by Tolbutamide and Diet Regulation', *Diabetes*, 29 (1980), 41–9.

8	Tuomilehto, J.,et.al & Finnish Diabetes Prevention Study Group (2001). Prevention of type 2 diabetes mellitus by changes in lifestyle among subjects with impaired glucose tolerance. *The New England journal of medicine*, 344(18), 1343–1350. https://doi.org/10.1056/NEJM200105033441801.

9	Eriksson, K. F., & Lindgärde, F. (1998). No excess 12-year mortality in men with impaired glucose tolerance who participated in the Malmö Preventive Trial with diet and exercise. *Diabetologia*, 41(9), 1010–1016. https://doi.org/10.1007/s001250051024

CHAPTER 2
# Fundamentals of Diabetes Prevention

Walking is man's best medicine.
**Hippocrates**

## Evidence in Diabetes Prevention

Several studies done in the past two decades have shown that diabetes is a preventable disease (**Table 2.1**). The earliest prevention trial was by Sartor et al. (1980). They studied 267 people with impaired glucose tolerance (IGT) in four arms—namely, diet, placebo, tolbutamide, and diet plus tolbutamide. They showed that those in the diet plus tolbutamide arm had lower progression to diabetes compared to the other arms.[1]

This triggered a flurry of studies that followed, including the Malmo Feasibility Study published in 1998, which showed that lifestyle modifications not only reduce the onset of diabetes among the IGT but also remitted early diabetes and improved metabolic profiles of these two groups, preventing cardiovascular complications.[2]

The Chinese Da Qing study published in 1997 was the largest prevention trial that studied 577 cohorts with IGT. Subjects were randomised into four groups—dieting and exercise, dieting alone, exercise alone, and control. The dietary arm received the luxury of customised food variations with personalised counselling and educational materials. The exercise group was asked to exercise according to individual quantified levels. The combined group was given both interventions. The diet alone arm was insignificant in reducing diabetes incidence, but the combined diet and exercise arm reduced diabetes by 31% compared with the control.[3]

The Finnish Diabetes Prevention Study (DPS) published in 2001 was another large study that followed the Da Qing study. It randomised 522 individuals with IGT into two arms, the intensive lifestyles plus dieting arm and the control arm with standard care. The interventional arm received individualised counselling, a circuit training programme, and regular follow-ups with dieting. This trial showed that intervention reduced diabetes by 58% compared with the control.[4]

The findings of diabetes prevention with intensive lifestyle modifications were supported by a bigger trial called the American Diabetes Prevention Program (DPP) published in 2002. This study recruited 3,234 subjects with prediabetes and divided them into three arms—lifestyle intervention and placebo, lifestyle intervention and metformin, and lifestyle intervention alone. In the intensive lifestyle arm, the cohorts were subjected to dieting, exercise (150 minutes/week with approximate weight loss of 7 to 10%), and behavioural modifications on a one-on-one basis with monthly reinforcement classes for individuals. It showed a reduction of diabetes by 58% in the intensive lifestyle management arm with the effect more pronounced in the lean elderly cohorts.[5]

The Indian Diabetes Prevention Program (IDPP) was another study that attempted to show that the application of intensive lifestyle modifications and drugs in reducing diabetes was consistent across geography and ethnicities with different physical attributes. It recruited 531 young lean Indians with IGT and followed them for thirty months and showed that lifestyle modification reduced diabetes by 28.5% and metformin by 26.4%, but there was no cumulative benefit.[6]

| Study | Publication Year | Intervention | | Cumulative Incidence % | RRR in the intervention arm (%) |
|---|---|---|---|---|---|
| Chinese Da Qing Study | 1997 | Exercise<br>Dieting<br>Exercise + Dieting<br>Control | 141<br>130<br>126<br>133 | 41.8<br>43.8<br>46<br>67.7 | 38 |
| Malmo Feasibility Study* | 1980 | Diet<br>Diet + Tolbutamide<br>Control | 98<br>49<br>120 | 13<br>0<br>29 | N/A<br>100 |
| Finnish DPPP | 2001 | Exercise + Dieting<br>Control | 265<br>257 | 10<br>22.95 | 58 |
| American DPPP | 2002 | Exercise + Dieting<br>Metformin<br>Control | 1079<br>1073<br>1082 | 14.7<br>21.7<br>28.9 | 58 |
| Indian DPPP | 2006 | Exercise + Dieting<br>Metformin<br>Lifestyle + Metformin<br>Control | 133<br>133<br>129<br>136 | 39.3<br>40.5<br>39.5<br>55 | 29 |
| STOP-NIDDM trial | 2002 | Acarbose<br>Control | 714<br>715 | 32<br>42 | 25 |
| Japanese Prevention Trial | 2004 | Exercise + Dieting<br>Control | 103<br>110 | 8.2<br>14.8 | 67 |

**Table 2.1** Summary of RCT in lifestyle treatment in the prevention of T2DM among the IFG.

N/A = not available.

*The Malmo study was not an RCT because the intervention group was not randomised.*

Reproduced from Kawa, L. (2022) Evidence in Primary Prevention of Type 2 Diabetes Mellitus—What It Means for Primary Prevention of Type 2 Diabetes Mellitus Epidemic in Papua New Guinea. *Journal of Diabetes Mellitus*, **12**, 87-97. doi: 10.4236/jdm.2022.122009.

Collectively, these studies showed that intensive lifestyle interventions can reduce/prevent high-risk individuals from developing diabetes. Furthermore, they showed that lifestyle intervention is effective across all multiracial and ethnic populations that span different geographies. However, there are no standardised dietary regimens from these studies. Moderate intensity exercises customised to individual patients for 30minutes per day is generally recommended.

> **Diabetes Prevention**
>
> 1. Intensive lifestyle change
> 2. Metformin prophylaxis

## Diabetes Prevention Strategies

T2DM is a preventable disease among the high-risk groups of various ethnicities from different geographies as shown by the large diabetes prevention studies.

The preventative strategies essentially fall under two main categories—pharmacological and non-pharmacological strategies.

### Pharmacological Strategy

Several pharmacological agents have also been studied in the prevention trials of diabetes (**Table 2.2**). Sartor et al., mentioned earlier, have shown that tolbutamide, a sulphonylureas, can be used with lifestyle intervention to reduce diabetes. They demonstrated that none of the patients on tolbutamide progressed to diabetes, compared with 29% in the control group.

The more robust American DPP showed that metformin, a biguanide oral hypoglycaemic agent, reduced overt diabetes in cohorts with IGT by 31%. The effect was more pronounced in younger cohorts with obesity. This was supported by the Indian DPP study, which reported a reduction of 26% in the metformin-treated arm compared to the placebo.

Acarbose, a glucosidase inhibitor of the small intestine, was also shown in the STOP NIDDM Trial (n=506) to reduce diabetes among the 221 cohorts with IGT by 32% compared to 285 cohorts who received placebo—a relative reduction of 10% compared to the controls. [7]

The Finnish DPP and the American DPP have shown that reduction of obesity as a risk factor for diabetes was associated with reduced incidence of diabetes among the high-risk group. This was followed up by the XENDOS study, which recruited normal glucose tolerance (NGT) and IGT (N=3305) obese individuals and randomised to lifestyle plus orlistat, a weight-reducing agent, or placebo. There was a 37% reduction in diabetes progression after five years, predominantly in the IGT group. [8]

Another class of drug called the glitazones was studied in several preventive trials. They all have shown significant reduction in diabetes among the high-risk groups. However, all the drugs were limited by significant side effects and intolerability. [9]

Drugs, therefore, have been shown to reduce diabetes incidences among the high-risk groups. However, none of these drugs except for metformin have been recommended for diabetes prevention by ADA since 2006. [10]

| Study | Publication Year | Intervention | | Cumulative Incidences (%) | RRR (%) |
|---|---|---|---|---|---|
| US DPP | 2002 | Metformin<br>Control | 1073<br>1082 | 21.7<br>28.9 | 31 |
| Indian DPP | 2006 | Metformin<br>Control | 133<br>136 | 40.5<br>55 | 26 |
| STOP NIDDM | 2002 | Acarbose<br>Control | 714<br>715 | 32<br>42 | 25 |
| Malmo Feasibility Study | 1980 | Tolbutamide<br>Control | | 0<br>29 | 100 |
| ACT-NOW | 2009 | Pioglitazone<br>Control | 213<br>228 | 3.1<br>8.2 | 81 |
| US DPP@ | 2005 | Troglitazone<br>Control | 585<br>582 | 30<br>35 | 45 |
| TRIPOD** | 1998 | Troglitazone<br>Control | 133<br>133 | 20<br>45 | 55 |
| DREAM | 2006 | Rosiglitazone<br>Control | 2635<br>2634 | 11.6<br>26 | 60 |

Table 2.2 A summary of RCT of pharmacotherapy in the prevention of diabetes among the IFG (High-Risk Group).

**33% attrition rate.*

*@ Incidence rates after Troglitazone withdrawal rose to similar levels as the placebo, and an inference was made that Troglitazone reduced diabetes.*

Reproduced from Kawa, L. (2022) Evidence in Primary Prevention of Type 2 Diabetes Mellitus—What It Means for Primary Prevention of Type 2 Diabetes Mellitus Epidemic in Papua New Guinea. *Journal of Diabetes Mellitus*, **12**, 87-97. doi: 10.4236/jdm.2022.122009.

### Non-pharmacological Strategy

All the landmark preventative trials mentioned before showed that lifestyle modifications by diet control and a supervised exercise regimen led to prevention of diabetes among high-risk groups in different ethnicities and geographical locations.

Dieting can be customised according to local varieties and availabilities. Supervised exercises produce more reduction in overt diabetes than the non–supervised exercises regimens. The American DPP study showed that exercise of at least 150 mins/week reduced diabetes by 7 to 10%. Therefore, the ADA recommends a minimum of 150 mins/week or 60 mins of brisk exercises thrice per week to benefit from diabetes reduction. [11]

**Diabetes Prevention Strategies**

1. Pharmacological
2. Non-pharmacological

- **Supervised exercise with dieting has maximal effect on preventing development of overt diabetes among the high-risk group and remits diabetes among those who already have diabetes .**
- **Aerobic exercise has maximal effect on prevention and remission.**
- **Metformin is the only approved drug used in prevention of diabetes among the high-risk group.**

## Types of Diabetes Prevention Approaches

The diabetes preventative strategies can be implemented in four different approaches among both the high-risk population and the population that has established diabetes. These four approaches are primary prevention, secondary prevention, tertiary prevention, and quaternary prevention .

**Four preventative approaches**

- Primary
- Secondary
- Tertiary
- Quaternary

### Primary Prevention

Strategies employed to prevent diabetes among those at high risk of developing diabetes are called primary prevention. These measures include pharmacological (metformin prophylaxis) and non-pharmacological lifestyle (dieting plus exercises) modifications.

The ADA in 2006 recommended metformin as the only diabetic drug for use as prophylaxis among the prediabetes patients. This recommendation stems from the Indian DPP trial that showed that the prediabetes group subjected to metformin had reduction of overt diabetes by 26.4%.

The US DPP showed that the prediabetes patients subjected to supervised exercise and dieting have better preventative outcomes compared with those who did not. Therefore, the minimum recommended exercise target is moderate exercise intensity for 150 minutes per week.

| Primary Prevention |
| --- |
| • Metformin prophylaxis<br>• Dieting and exercise |

## Secondary Prevention

The preventative approaches employed in preventing acute and chronic complications among patients already having established diabetes are called secondary prevention. These include both pharmacological and non-pharmacological measures underpinned by intensive glycaemic control with optimal management of other conventional cardiovascular risk factors to target.

| Secondary Prevention |
| --- |
| • Set target HBA1c customised to patient and work to achieve it within three to six months.<br>• Start ACE-I/ARB for BP control to target or CCB if contraindicated.<br>• Start statin or cholesterol therapy and treat to target.<br>• Continue primary prevention. |

## Tertiary Prevention

The approaches involved in managing complications of patients having established diabetes to prevent early morbidity and mortality are called tertiary prevention. This is underpinned by customising glycaemic control as per the ADA/EASD 2012 Consensus Statement. [12]

| Tertiary Prevention |
| --- |
| • Customise or personalise glycaemic control.<br>• Customise exercise therapy according to presence and/or absence of complications.<br>• Customise management of chronic complications:<br>  ▪ Phototherapy of retina if neovascularisation<br>  ▪ Appropriate heart failure management<br>  ▪ Podotherapy for neuropathic or arteriopathic ulcers<br>  ▪ Appropriate management of neuropathies (autonomic, peripheral, and mononeuropathies)<br>  ▪ Appropriate renal therapy with consideration of early RRT in stage IV CRF and complications of renal failure<br>  ▪ Phosphodiesterase therapy for erectile dysfunction<br>  ▪ Insulin dose adjustments in those with labile blood glucose (BG). If uncontrolled, consider continuous insulin pumps (CSIIP). |

## Quaternary Prevention

This strategy involves prevention of 'over-medicalisation', of diabetic patients and is often termed the 'prevention of polypharmacy'

The inherent risk of over-medicalisation is where many drugs can potentially be prescribed without evidence. The healthcare provider (HCP) needs to ensure patients are prescribed appropriate medicines based on evidence and as and when required and cease any other medications not required.

---

- **Primary prevention is prevention of diabetes through lifestyle changes and metformin prophylaxis among those at high risk.**
- **Secondary prevention is prevention of complications of diabetes underlined by optimal glycaemic control.**
- **Tertiary prevention is retarding the progression of the complications in organs to end stages and death underpinned by personalised glycaemic control. It is the control of complications**
- **Quaternary prevention is the prevention of polypharmacy in diabetic patients.**

---

# Screening for Diabetes

Diabetes is a chronic disease with complications that impose enormous direct and indirect economic, social, and health costs on the healthcare system and individuals worldwide. Although, screening could be expensive in some aspects, screening with a view to prevention reduces these costs in the long term.

## Wilson and Jungner's Criteria for Screening

For any disease or condition to qualify for screening, the Wilson and Jungner criteria must be met. These criteria include:

- The disease should be an important health problem.
- The disease should have an early asymptomatic phase.
- The disease should have an effective screening test.
- The disease should have an available effective treatment.
- There should be evidence that early treatment of asymptomatic patients improves outcomes.

Diabetes mellitus meets all these criteria and, therefore, qualifies to be screened. Screening for Type 1 diabetes mellitus (T1DM) is not recommended even though it meets the Wilson and Junger's screening criteria. Although, the immune markers (ICA, IAA, GAD, IA-2) in T1DM individuals suggest a population at risk of developing T1DM, they are not used as screening tools because of the following reasons: there are no treatment when the antibodies are positive, it is costly to screen given the low incidence of T1DM and the cut-off marks are not established.

## Types of Screening Strategies

There are three types of screening strategies for diabetes. The type employed depends on the objective and the availability of resources. They include

a. *Population or Community Screening*
   This type of screening involving the whole population is expensive, tedious, and requires a lot of time and resources.

b.  *Targeted or Selective Screening*
    This is screening of a subgroup of patients identified as at high risk for developing T2DM.

c.  *Opportunistic Screening*
    Screening of patients for diabetes who present to health care institutions or at any point of care for reasons other than diabetes is very easy, cheap, and requires minimal manpower and resources than the other two types of screening.

---

**Three Types of Diabetes Screening**

- Population (community) screening
- Targeted or selective screening
- Opportunistic screening

---

## Screening Tools

Screening for diabetes can be done with any one of the following tools:

- *Capillary blood glucose*, while less sensitive than other screening tools, is cheap and readily available. Those with higher glucose can be subjected to a plasma glucose, either fasting or prandial, two hours after last meal.
- *Oral glucose tolerance test (OGTT)* is recommended by WHO for screening and diagnostic purpose. It is, however, more expensive, less reproducible, and more inconvenient than capillary blood glucose testing.
- *HBA1c* testing is easy and reproducible but more expensive than the capillary and the OGTT and is not readily available.

## Screening Frequency

The frequency of screening for diabetes depends on the age and the presence or absence of the risk factors for diabetes. The ADA recommends that those without the risk factors be tested at the age of forty-five years and then every three years. Those with BMI of ≥25 kgm$^2$ and with ≥1 risk factors should be screened earlier and every three years.

## Screening for High-Risk Population

Screening is an essential approach to prevention of T2DM. There is no evidence of benefits from screening asymptomatic individuals for T2DM.[13] However, there is overwhelming consensus among experts that screening is essential for diagnosis and prevention of diabetes among the high-risk population. The subgroup of patients categorised as high risk for developing diabetes are those with the following risk factors:

- Ethnicity
  In the United Kindom, the Southeast Asian population (Indians, Pakistanis, Bangladeshis, and Sri Lankans) are deemed the high-risk ethnic group. In PNG, the Wanigelas and the Tolais were intiallly deemed high risk. Today, everyone in PNG who has other risk factors are at high risk for developing T2DM.

- Positive family history of diabetes
- Metabolic syndrome
- Obesity
- Prediabetes (impaired fasting blood glucose, impaired glucose tolerance test)
- Gestational diabetes
- HBA1c of 5.7 - 6.4

## Diabetes Risks Assessment and Stratifications

The Framingham risk tool is a primary preventative risk engine that has been used for decades to assess and stratify risks of cardiovascular disease for both diabetes and non-diabetes patients without cardiovascular disease. The modified version in 2000 has removed diabetes and assigned it as myocardial equivalent, meaning diabetes is equivalent to having an MI, requiring aggressive management of glycaemia and the conventional cardiovascular risk factors reduction.

### The Framingham Risk Score

This score assesses the probability of CVE in ten years, and this is given as follows:

- Low risk (<10% risk after ten years)—82% of patients
- Intermediate risk (10–20% risk after ten years)—16% of patients
- High risk (>20% risk in ten years)—3% of patients

### The QRISK Score

The QRISK is a secondary risk score validated in the United Kingdom and currently recommended for assessing cardiovascular risk among the established diabetes patients. The ASSIGN risk calculator is the Scottish version, and these calculators can be accessed online for assessing cardiovascular risks among T2DM patients.

### CV Risk Assessment Tools

- Framingham score
- QRISK score / ASSIGN risk calculators

## Key Messages:

- **Supervised exercise and dieting have maximal effect on diabetes prevention.**
- **Metformin can be used as chemoprophylaxis for those with prediabetes.**
- **Diabetes meets the criteria for screening among those with high risks for prevention.**
- **The type of screening strategy employed is dependent on the availability of resources, the population at risk, and the prevalence.**
- **Risk tools are available online for assessment of diabetic risks for development of cardiovascular diseases**

# References:

1   Sartor G, Schersten B, Carlstrom S. et al. Ten-year follow-up of subjects with impaired glucose tolerance. Prevention of diabetes by tolbutamide and diet regulation. Diabetes 1980; 29, 41-9. https://doi.org/10.2337/diabetes.29.1.41

2   K. F. Eriksson and F. Lindgarde, 'No Excess 12-Year Mortality in Men with Impaired Glucose Tolerance Who Participated in the Malm¨o Preventive Trial with Diet and Exercise', *Diabetologia* 41 (1998), 1,010–16.

3   Pan, X. et.al., (1997). Effects of diet and exercise in preventing NIDDM in people with impaired glucose tolerance. The Da Qing IGT and Diabetes Study. *Diabetes care, 20*(4), 537–544. https://doi.org/10.2337/diacare.20.4.537.

4   Tuomilehto J, Lindstr̈om J, Erisson JG, Valle TT, Hämäläinen H, Ilanne-Parikka P, et al. Finnish Diabetes Prevention Study Group. Prevention of type 2 diabetes mellitus by changes in lifestyle among subjects with impaired glucose tolerance. N Engl J Med 2001; 344(18):1343-50.https://doi.org/10.1056/NEJM200105033441801

5   Knowler, et.al., & Diabetes Prevention Program Research Group (2002). Reduction in the incidence of type 2 diabetes with lifestyle intervention or metformin. *The New England journal of medicine, 346*(6), 393–403. https://doi.org/10.1056/NEJMoa012512.

6   Ramachandran, A., Snehalatha, C., Mary, S., Mukesh, B., Bhaskar, A. D., Vijay, V., & Indian Diabetes Prevention Programme (IDPP) (2006). The Indian Diabetes Prevention Programme shows that lifestyle modification and metformin prevent type 2 diabetes in Asian Indian subjects with impaired glucose tolerance (IDPP-1). *Diabetologia, 49*(2), 289–297. https://doi.org/10.1007/s00125-005-0097-z.

7   Chiasson, J. L., Josse, R. G., Gomis, R., Hanefeld, M., Karasik, A., Laakso, M., & STOP-NIDDM Trail Research Group (2002). Acarbose for prevention of type 2 diabetes mellitus: the STOP-NIDDM randomised trial. *Lancet (London, England), 359*(9323), 2072–2077. https://doi.org/10.1016/S0140-6736(02)08905-5.

8   Chiasson, J. L., Josse, R. G., Gomis, R., Hanefeld, M., Karasik, A., Laakso, M., & STOP-NIDDM Trail Research Group (2002). Acarbose for prevention of type 2 diabetes mellitus: the STOP-NIDDM randomised trial. *Lancet (London, England), 359*(9323), 2072–2077. https://doi.org/10.1016/S0140-6736(02)08905-5.

9   DeFronzo, R.A., Tripathy, D., Schwenke, D.C., Banerji, M., Bray, G.A., Buchanan, T.A., Clement, S.C., Henry, R.R., Hodis, H.N., Kitabchi, A.E...., and ACT NOW Study group. Pioglitazone for di-abetes prevention in impaired glucose tolerance. N Engl J Med. 2011; 364: 1104-1115. https://doi.org/10.1056/NEJMoa1010949

10  Nathan DM, Davidson M, DeFronzo RA et al. Impaired Fasting Glucose and Impaired Glucose Tolerance: Implications for Care. A Consensus Statement from the American Diabetes Association. Diabetes Care 2007; 30: 753-9.https://doi.org/10.2337/dc07-9920

11  American Diabetes Association. http://www.diabetes.org/food-and-fitness/fitness/physical- activity-is-important.html

12  Inzucchi, S. E., Bergenstal, R. M., Buse, J. B.,et. al., (2012). Management of hyperglycaemia in type 2 diabetes: a patient-centered approach. Position statement of the American Diabetes Association (ADA) and the European Association for the Study of Diabetes (EASD). *Diabetologia, 55*(6), 1577–1596. https://doi.org/10.1007/s00125-012-2534-0

13  Engelgau, M. M., Aubert, R. E., Thompson, T. J., & Herman, W. H. (1995). Screening for NIDDM in nonpregnant adults. A review of principles, screening tests, and recommendations. *Diabetes care, 18*(12), 1606–1618. https://doi.org/10.2337/diacare.18.12.1606

# CHAPTER 3
# Diagnosis and Classification of Diabetes

*Man may be the captain of his fate, but he is also the victim of his blood sugar.*
**Wilfrid G. Oakley**

## Diagnosis of Diabetes Mellitus

The words *diabetes* and *mellitus* are derived from Greek and Latin respectively. Diabetes, in Greek, means to siphon — 'to pass through'—and mellitus, in Latin, means 'honey' or sweet because excess sugar was noted in urine.[1] In fact, tasting urine was the first method of diagnosis of diabetes, used since 1700 until blood testing became available in the 1960s.[2]

The diagnosis of diabetes today is essentially blood based and these include:

- *Capillary blood glucose*, which is readily available and cheap. It is, however, used only as a screening tool for symptomatic and asymptomatic patients and for self-monitoring of blood glucose among those who have diabetes. It is not used for diagnostic purposes.
- *Plasma venous blood*—both random and fasting blood glucose are used for diagnosis.
- *Oral glucose tolerance test*, which is recommended by the WHO for diagnosis of diabetes among the asymptomatic and gestational diabetes.
- *HBA1c*, recommended by WHO for diagnosing T2DM but is not recommended in diagnosing T1DM.

| Diagnostic criterion | WHO | ADA |
|---|---|---|
| Fasting plasma glucose | ≥7mmol/L | ≥7 mmol/L |
| Random plasma glucose | ≥11.1mmol/L | ≥ 11.1mmol/L |
| HBA1c | ≥ 6.5% | ≥6.5% |
| 2-Hrs OGTT | ≥11.1mmol/L | ≥11.1 mmol/L |

Table 3.1 Diabetes diagnostic criteria. Reproduced from World Health Organization (WHO) and American Diabetes Association (ADA), 2006.

### WHO Diabetes Diagnostic Criteria

Diabetes is diagnosed today using the WHO diagnostic (clinical and blood testing) criteria.

- Symptomatic patients (polyuria, polydipsia, polyphagia, weight loss) plus random blood glucose ≥ 11.1 mmol/L or fasting blood glucose ≥7 mmol/L or oral glucose tolerance test ≥ 11.1mmol/L.
- Asymptomatic patients RBSL ≥11.1 mmol/L, 2-hr prandial glucose ≥11.1mmol/L. Asymptomatic patients with one abnormal blood sugar test need a repeat test to confirm diabetes.
- HBA1c ≥6.5%

> ### WHO Diagnostic Criteria for Diabetes Mellitus
>
> 1. Symptomatic with either RBSL ≥11.1mmol/l or FBSL ≥7mmol/l or two-hour prandial glucose ≥ 11.1mmol/l
> 2. Asymptomatic patients must have two blood tests (RBSL or FBSL) at different times to confirm diabetes.
> 3. Two-hour OGTT 11.1mmo/l or HBA1c ≥6.5%

## Diagnosis of Prediabetes

The term 'prediabetes' is a generic term that is used to describe the state between normal glycaemia and diabetes. It includes two different entities known as the impaired fasting glucose (IFG) and the impaired glucose tolerance (IGT).

The two states of prediabetes have different definitions, prevalence, pathophysiology, and risks of progression into overt diabetes[3] which can generally take years.

Different literatures state different prevalence rates between 25 and 70%. The natural history of the prediabetes suggests that, 25% convert to overt diabetes, 50% remain in the prediabetes states, and 25% revert to normoglycemic state.

### Impaired Fasting Glucose (IFG)

IFG is defined as elevation of fasting glucose ≥ 5.6 to 6.9 mmol/L. It has a prevalence of approximately 26%, and its underlying pathophysiology is hepatic insulin resistance, where early insulin action (0 to 10 minutes) is impaired.

### Impaired Glucose Tolerance (IGT)

IGT is defined as glucose ≥ 7.8 mmol/L to 11.1 mmol/L after two hours 75 g OGTT. It has a prevalence of 15% and varies between different ethnic groups. It is noted to be due to the late (60 to 120 minutes) insulin resistance in the muscle.

> ### Prediabetes
>
> • IFG and IGT are states between normal glycemia and diabetes.
> • They differ in definitions, diagnostic criteria, pathophysiology, risks of conversion to overt diabetes, and prevalence

| Diagnostic Criterion | WHO | ADA | NICE |
|---|---|---|---|
| Fasting plasma glucose | 6.1 – 6.9mmol/L | 5.6 – 6.9mmol/L | 6.1 – 6.9mmol/L |
| 2- hour OGTT | 7.8 – 11.0mmol/L | 7.8 – 11.0mmol/L | 7.8 – 11.0mmol/L |
| HBA1c | 6 – 6.4% | 5.7 – 6.4% | 6 – 6.4% |

**Table 3.2** Diagnostic criteria for prediabetes by different organisations: WHO = World Health Organisation, ADA = American Diabetes Association, NICE = National Institute Clinical Excellence, OGTT = Oral Glucose Tolerance Test.

The WHO and the ADA recommend different diagnostic thresholds for prediabetes, which can be confusing. The ADA diagnostic criteria reduce the threshold of diagnosis compared with the WHO criteria as shown in **Table 3.2**. The implications for this mean that the ADA criteria would include more people diagnosed as prediabetes and, thus, require more resources and efforts in their management compared with the WHO and NICE criteria.[4] However, the earlier the detection, the greater the preventative efforts that could be put in place to reduce transition to overt diabetes.

The diagnostic criteria published by the WHO in 2006 is generally accepted by many countries and organisations, including the IDF and the Diabetes UK.[5]

**Two Prediabetes Stages**

1. Impaired fasting glucose (IFG)
2. Impaired glucose tolerance (IGT)

## Formation and Roles of Glycated Haemoglobin A1c (HBA1c)

### Glycation (Formation)

The glucose in the blood reacts spontaneously with the NH2 amino acid terminal of the beta side chain of human haemoglobin and forms the HBA1c in a ketoamine linkage. This process is called 'glycation'. HBA1c is easier to measure than the other minor components that appear to be adducts of products of glucose-6 phosphate and fructose 1-6 phosphate. They are slowly and continuously formed throughout the 120-day life cycle of the red blood cells. In diabetic patients, these normal reactions increase two to threefold.[6]

### Diagnostic Tool

The potential role of HBA1c as a diagnostic tool was mentioned in 1985. The ADA proposed HBA1c ≥6.5% for diagnosis of type 2 diabetes in 2005. However, the WHO and IDF joint expert committee felt there was insufficient evidence for acceptance. The International Expert Committee Report in 2009, with further evidence, gave credence to the suggestion, but the WHO did not approve HBA1c as a diagnostic tool until in 2011.[7]

## Therapeutic Tool

HbA1c is now primarily used to assess glycaemic control among the diabetic patients already on treatment over a three-month period. This allows physicians to optimise antidiabetic treatment. [7]

## Prognostic Tool

The role of HBA1c has expanded recently from being a mere surrogate for glycaemic control to a diagnostic criterion for diabetes. It could now be potentially used as a prognostic marker among patients with long-standing diabetes as shown in the ACCORD trial.

The ACCORD trial looked at intensive versus standard treatment but among a different population (elderly with long-standing diabetes and multiple comorbidities). This trial showed the intensive arm with HBA1c 6.4% was associated with 22% increase in all-cause mortality. [8]

This mortality was concentrated in a subgroup of patients who did not achieve >0.5% reduction of HBA1c from baseline above 7.5%. It appears that continuing to seek HBA1c <7% may be hazardous and a target range of 7 to 8% may be appropriate to this patient population.

There is a suggestion that, if patients are followed up for three to four months and found to have no drop in HBA1c by 0.5% from baseline, this could suggest a high-risk group. Advice is that these patients' HBA1c must not be reduced with aggressive treatment but maintained above 7%

> ### Roles of HBA1c in Diabetes Medicine
>
> - Monitoring of glycaemic control
> - Diagnostic criteria
> - Prognostic criteria

## Issues with HBA1c

There are several issues clinicians must take into consideration when interpreting HBA1c tests:

- HBA1c is reduced in the following conditions:
  - Patients taking iron and vitamin B12 supplements
  - Liver disease
  - High red cell turn-over, for example in thalassemia and malaria with haemolysis
- HBA1c is increased in the following conditions:
  - Chronic renal failure
  - Alcoholism
  - Patients taking aspirin

It is not recommended to diagnose DM in pregnant women, children, adolescents, and those with T1DM.

## Classification of Diabetes

The classification of diabetes has evolved over time from a therapeutic-based classification to that of both treatment and etiological-based classifications.

The first diabetes classification was released in 1977 by the National Diabetes Data Group. [9] This classification was based on the type of treatment for diabetes and included the following:

- Insulin-dependent diabetes mellitus (IDDM)
- Non-insulin-dependent diabetes mellitus (NIDDM)
- Gestational diabetes mellitus
- Malnutrition-related diabetes mellitus
- Other types of diabetes

Two further reviews of the classification were conducted in 1982 and 1987. The recent review gives an etiological-based classification. In addition, the new classification acknowledges the heterogeneity of the metabolic glucose disturbances in the clinical presentation. This classification is as follows:

1. **Type 1 Diabetes Mellitus (T1DM)**
   a. *Type 1a (immune-mediated insulinopenia)*
      Most patients with T1DM have this form (90%), characterised by the presence of the autoantibodies to the islet cells or the insulin and its receptors.

   b. *Type 1b (idiopathic insulinopenia)*
      This type is characterised by permanent insulinopenia without any evidence of autoimmunity. It is less common (10%) than the immune-mediated form and is commonly seen in African and Asian cohorts. There is strong suggestion of inheritance.

2. **Type 2 Diabetes Mellitus (T2DM)**
   The pathogenesis of T2DM is on a continuum. It ranges from insulin secretory defect to relative resistance to insulin and absolute insulin resistance.

3. **Other Diabetes**
   This group includes diabetes caused by rare genetic abnormalities affecting the beta cells and insulin action, which are beyond the scope of this book for further explanation.

### Genetic Defects of Beta Cells

Diabetes related to genetic defects of the beta cells are commonly known as the maturity onset diabetes of the young (MODY), are seen in those who are less than 45 years, who have absence of ßeta cell autoimmunity, absence of insulin resistance, progressive impairment of insulin secretion with minimal or no defects in the insulin action (**Figure 3.1**). These types are also known as 'monogenic diabetes' to distinguish them from the most common T1DM and T2DM, which are influenced by more complex genetic and environmental factors.

They demonstrate autosomal dominant inheritance and affect the first and the second generations of family lines. There is initial insulin secretion, but that declines as patients grow older. The clinical presentations vary extensively among patients. Initially, patients require oral hypoglycaemic therapy with sulfonylureas which controls the sugar ('Honeymoon period'), but ultimately, they end up insulinopenic requiring insulin. [10] Six of these gene defects are:

- MODY 1 defect in HNF-4a gene
- MODY 2 defect in glucokinase gene
- MODY 3 defect in HFN-1a gene
- MODY 4 defect in IPF-1 gene
- MODY 5 defect in HNF-1b
- MODY 6 defect in neuroD1 gene

MODY 1 patients are usually born with high birthweight (app. 4kgs) and note to be hypoglycaemic. MODY 2 have a prevalence of 30 – 50% and have a milder form of diabetes. They are usually detected incidentally and rarely develop chronic complications. MODY 3 is the most common type among patients with European ancestry (50 – 70%). They tend to respond to sulphonylureas and have low renal glucose thresholds. MODY 5 may have associated renal cysts, uterine abnormalities, and gout.

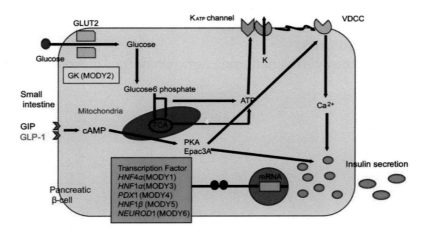

**Figure 3.1** The genetic defects in the genes causing MODY leads to beta cell destruction with impaired production and secretion of insulin. Urakami T. Maturity-onset diabetes of the young (MODY): current perspectives on diagnosis and treatment. *'Diabetes, Metabolic Syndrome and Obesity: Targets and Therapy 2019:12 1047-1056'* Originally published by and reproduced with permission from Dove Medical Press Ltd.

## Genetic Defects in Insulin Action

Rare and unusual causes of diabetes resulting from genetic defects in abnormalities of insulin action. Three types in these subgroups are noted:

- Type A insulin resistance
- Leprechaunism syndrome
- Rabson–Mendelhall syndrome

4. **Disease of Exocrine Pancreases**
   Any pathological processes that affect the pancreas have the potential to cause diabetes. Most pancreatic diseases are acquired and include infections, trauma, pancreatectomy, and fibro calculous pancreatopathy.

5. **Endocrinopathies**

   Supraphysiological levels of insulin-antagonising hormones (GH, cortisol, glucagon, and epinephrine) can cause diabetes. Fortunately, this type of diabetes is curable when the underlying hormonal abnormality is rectified.

6. **Drug- or Chemical-Induced Diabetes Mellitus**

   Many drugs can either cause or precipitate diabetes in insulin-resistance individuals.

7. **Infections**

   Infections leading to destructions of the beta cells can potentially cause diabetes. Examples includes congenital rubella, CMV, adenovirus, and Coxsackie virus.

8. **Genetic Syndromes Associated with Diabetes**

   Several genetic syndromes are associated with diabetes. These include Down syndrome, Klinefelter's syndrome, Turner's syndrome, and Wolfram's syndrome.

9. **Gestational Diabetes Mellitus (GDM)**

   GDM is defined as glucose intolerance with the onset or on first recognition during pregnancy.

10. **Prediabetes States (IGT/IFG)**

    IGT/IFG is defined as the intermediate state between normal glucose homeostasis and diabetes.

---

### Two Types of Diabetes Classifications

1. Treatment-based classification
2. Pathological (etiological) classification

---

## Heterogeneity of Diabetes

The traditional categorisation of diabetes defines two types, either as T1DM or T2DM. However, recently, certain diabetes has been noted to behave like neither of these two traditional classes. These forms of diabetes are called the 'Hybrid diabetes'. They have contemporary therapeutic and prognostic challenges. The four hybrid forms are described in the following sections.

### Latent Autoimmune Diabetes in Adult (LADA)

This is a slow-burning variant of T1DM that is characterised by the presence of autoantibodies. However, it has a natural history of slow progression to ultimate insulin dependency by 30 to 35 years of age. Unlike the classical T1DM, which presents with insulin dependency earlier, LADA patients are treated with oral hypoglycaemic agents until later in the duration ('Honeymoon period'). This could be difficult to differentiate from T2DM.[11]

## Maturity Onset Diabetes of the Young (MODY)

This hybrid form of diabetes is due to the genetic defects of beta cells where there is impaired insulin secretion with minimal or no defect in insulin action. It is transmitted as autosomal dominant with first, second, and even third generations affected. It is diagnosed among young patients under 25 years of age. [12]

## Ketosis Prone Diabetes (KPD)

Ketosis and ketonuria were predominantly associated more with T1DM than T2DM. Recent findings that T1DM or T2DM can be either or neither of them has further blurred the classification. Diagnosis of this category of hybrid diabetes is by the Aß (**a**utoantibody, **b**eta cell function) system. [13]

- A+ß-. Autoantibodies present, β cell function absent (54%)
- A+ß+. Autoantibodies present, β cell function present (8%)
- A-ß-. Autoantibodies absent, β cell function absent (20%)
- A-ß+. Autoantibodies absent, β cell function present (18%

## Type 2 Diabetes Mellitus in Children

More children are now being diagnosed with T2DM in concordance with the rising epidemic of childhood obesity today than before.

| *Hybrid Forms of Diabetes* |
| --- |
| <ul><li>Latent autoimmune diabetes of adult (LADA)</li><li>Maturity onset diabetes of the young (MODY)</li><li>Ketosis prone diabetes (KPD)</li><li>Type 2 diabetes in children</li></ul> |

## Key Messages:

- **Diagnosis of diabetes is based on WHO diagnostic criteria characterised by symptoms of glucotoxicity and plasma glucose and HBA1c level.**
- **Prediabetes is a high-risk state between normoglycemia and diabetes with different pathophysiology and natural history.**
- **HBA1c is now used as a tool for diagnosis of diabetes, treatment of diabetes and monitoring of glycaemic control. It can also be considered as a prognostic tool.**
- **The new diabetes classification is etiologically based.**
- **Hybrid diabetes have now blurred the treatment-based classification of diabetes as T1DM and T2DM.**

# References:

1    Mandal A. History of Diabetes. https://www.news-medical.net/health/History-of-Diabetes

2    Diabetes UK. History of Diabetes. https://www.diabetes.co.uk/diabetes-history.

3    Nathan, D. M., Davidson, M. B., DeFronzo, R. A. et.al, & American Diabetes Association (2007). Impaired fasting glucose and impaired glucose tolerance: implications for care. *Diabetes care, 30*(3), 753–759. https://doi.org/10.2337/dc07-9920.

4    *Definition and Diagnosis of Diabetes Mellitus and the Intermediate Hyperglycaemia (2006). A Report of a WHO/IDF Consultation.* https://www.who.int./publication/i/item/definition-and-diagnosis-of-diabetes-mellitus-intermediate-hyperglycemia.

5    Diabetes UK. The New Diagnostic Criteria for Diabetes. https://www.diabetes.org.uk/Professional/Position-statements-reports/Diagnosis-ongoing management-monitoring.

6    Bunn, H. F., Gabbay, K. H., & Gallop, P. M. (1978). The glycosylation of haemoglobin: relevance to diabetes mellitus. *Science (New York, N.Y.), 200*(4337), 21–27. https://doi.org/10.1126/science.635569.

7    *Use of Glycated Haemoglobin (HbA1c) in the Diagnosis of Diabetes Mellitus: Abbreviated Report of a WHO Consultation.* (2011). World Health Organization.

8    Action to Control Cardiovascular Risk in Diabetes Study Group, Gerstein, H. C., Miller, M. E., Byington, R. P.et. al.,(2008). Effects of intensive glucose lowering in type 2 diabetes. *The New England journal of medicine, 358*(24), 2545–2559. https://doi.org/10.1056/NEJMoa0802743

9    Diabetes mellitus. Report of a WHO Study Group. (1985). *World Health Organization technical report series, 727,* 1–113.

10   Mcphee S, Papadakis M & Rabow M. *Lange Current Medical Diagnosis and Treatment* (Mc Graw Hill, 2011).

11   Kumar P, Clark M. *Kumar & Clark's Clinical Medicine*, 7th edn (Saunders, 2009).

12   Genuth, S., Alberti, K. G., Bennett, P.et.al.& Expert Committee on the Diagnosis and Classification of Diabetes Mellitus (2003). Follow-up report on the diagnosis of diabetes mellitus. *Diabetes care, 26*(11), 3160–3167. https://doi.org/10.2337/diacare.26.11.3160

13   Ketosis Prone Diabetes Mellitus. Medscape Medicine. https://www.emedicine.medscape.com/article/215425-medication.

# CHAPTER 4
# Management of Diabetes

The three pillars of diabetes medicine are: dieting, exercise, and pharmacotherapy.
**Elliot Joslin**

Diabetes was a fatal condition prior to the discovery of insulin in 1921. Since then, advancements have been made to refine and modify the insulin molecule more suitable for treatment of diabetes. The newer insulins with better efficacy, duration, and safety profiles were engineered and produced en masse and with the refining of the treatment strategies, survival of diabetics has reached near normal level. Thus, diabetes outcome has been improved by the discovery and the refining of insulin from being a fatal condition to a chronic treatable condition.

There are three current pillars of diabetes management—diet, exercise, and pharmacological treatments.

## Lifestyle Modification Therapy

Dieting and exercise make up two of the three pillars of diabetic management. Recent large preventative trials discussed in chapter 2, have shown that introducing both dieting and exercise among those at high risk of developing diabetes in different ethnicities from different geographies have led to the prevention of diabetes. Further, these preventative trials have also been shown to control glycaemia and even remit diabetes in those who had established diabetes.

### Dieting Prescription

Although dieting is prescribed for all the prediabetes and the diabetes patients, there are no standardised dietary regimens. Further, diet alone has been equivocal in diabetes prevention. However, combining dietary changes with exercises have been shown to be more effective than the diet changes alone.

### Exercise Prescription

Recent studies have shown that prescribed exercise regimens do prevent diabetes among the prediabetes and remit those with the established diabetes. Supervised exercise prescription further improves other cardiovascular risk factors such as weight loss, reduction in blood pressure, lipids, and the general well-being of patients. This has led to the concept of 'exercise prescription' for those at high risk of diabetes and those with established diabetes.

Exercise prescription is to be preceded by a premedical assessment to establish the physical status and the abilities of the patients as many diabetics have many physical limitations and disabilities incurred by the diabetes complications and other associated comorbidities. [1]

Exercise prescription is then tailored according to the patient's need and delivered slowly and in a more acclimatised manner. Both the aerobic and the resistance categories of exercises can be prescribed with maximal benefits accrued when combined and closely supervised.

**Combined dieting and exercise prescription lead to 58% reduction in diabetes. Metformin plus lifestyle modification leads to 32% reduction.**

## Pre-Exercise Medical Assessment

The ADA and the American College of Sports Medicine (ACSM) have jointly recommended pre-exercise medical assessment of diabetic patients before prescribing exercise treatment.[1] This is because diabetes patients have more disabilities that impair exercise and even predispose patients to deterioration of complications—including premature deaths from cardiovascular diseases—compared with non-diabetic populations.[2] For example, people with peripheral neuropathy risk fractures and trauma of the foot, if engaged in weight-bearing and high-impact exercises such as running. They would require appropriate size footwear with low- to moderate-intensity exercises on flat surfaces. Proliferative diabetic retinopathic patients risk retinal detachments and vitreous haemorrhage when engaged in moderate- to high-intensity resistance exercises and patients with autonomic neuropathy have high risk of adverse cardiovascular outcomes when subjected to moderate- to high-intensity exercises. Therefore, understanding patients' morbidity and status from a pre-exercise medical assessment is a pre-requisite to prescribing exercise regimens. In addition, this is done as an individualised approach to allow patients to develop tolerance and to reduce undue complications and derive maximal benefits.

The American Heart Association (AHA) has released its own recommendations for the pre-exercise assessment of diabetic patients in those with cardiovascular risk factors who have high risk for adverse cardiovascular outcomes when subjected to moderate- to high-intensity exercises. Those with known CAD undergo supervised evaluation of ischemic response to exercise and arrhythmic risk before exercise.[3]

**Lifestyle management of diabetes involves the following in order of priority:**

- **Pre-medical assessment for presence and/or absence of complications and limitations**
- **Dietary and exercise prescriptions**

## Pharmacotherapy

Pharmacological treatment is the third pillar of treatment of diabetes and in the centre of this pillar lies the insulin. Insulin remains the foundation of pharmacotherapy of diabetes. It is now used to treat both the T1DM and the T2DM with great success.

Many other new oral and injectables pharmacotherapies have been added onto the armamentarium of drugs against diabetes over the decades.

### Treatment Modalities of Diabetes

- Dieting
- Exercises
- Drug

## Traditional Therapies

Pharmacotherapy in diabetes is a dynamic field that continues to churn out new drugs into the market. The traditional therapies currently in use include the followings:

- Sulphonylureas
- Biguanide
- Glitazones
- Acarbose
- Insulins (short and the intermediate-acting insulins).

### Sulphonylureas

Sulfonylurea is a group of drugs with well-known glucose lowering effects. They stimulate insulin release by blocking the ATP sensitive potassium channels on the Beta cells, reducing potassium permeability. This reduces the positive charge in the Beta cell causing influx of calcium through the L-type $Ca^{2+}$ channel which cause the depolarization that facilitates insulin secretion.[4] (**Figure 4.1**). They are classed as second-line drugs on the ADA/EASD treatment guidelines.

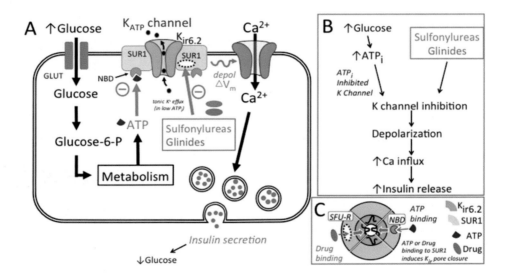

**Figure 4.1** Mechanism of Sulfonylurea. Reproduced with permission from PharmWiki, Tulane University School of Medicine.

The sulphonylureas only work in those with preserved or remaining Beta cell function but do not work in those with absent and or declining beta cell functions. They induce insulin release in a glucose-independent manner meaning that regardless of plasma glucose level, sulphonylureas will continue to *stimulate* insulin secretion. This has the tendency to cause hypoglycaemia in those with low plasma glucose.

They have a decelerating effect on the glycaemic control. This means that they have good glycaemic control in the first three months, followed by reduction of their effects in the next three months by 50%. The sulphonylureas are no longer effective after six months.

Recent studies suggest that binding of the sulphonylureas on the myocardial ATP sensitive potassium channels could mechanistically attenuate the 'ischemic preconditioning', a protective mechanism of myocardium against significant myocardial damage from ischemic heart disease.[5]

They are classified into three generations depending on their chronology.

## First generation

- Tolbutamide
- Tolazamide
- Chlorpropamide
- Acetohexamide

## Second generation

- Glibenclamide
- Gliclazide
- Glipizide
- Glyclopyramide

## Third generation

- Glimepiride—often considered as second generation

### Biguanide

Metformin is the only biguanide in use today in the management of T2DM. It is now considered the first-line therapy in T2DM and appears to exert some metabolic effects on patients with abdominal obesity and IFG.

Its mechanism of action is to reduce gluconeogenesis from the liver, decrease glycogenolysis, facilitate glucose disposal into peripheral tissues, reduce fatty acid oxidation, and protect the cardiovascular system from the negative effects of hyperglycaemia.[6] (**Figure 4.2**)

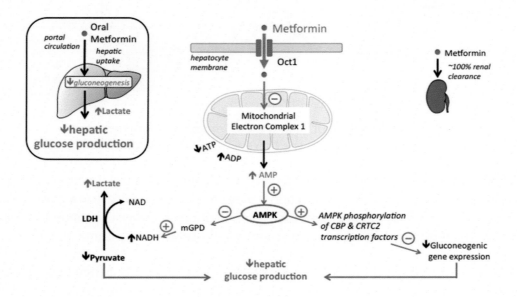

**Figure 4.2.** Mechanism of metformin. Metformin, absorbed from the gut through the portal vein, enters the hepatocyte via Oct1 receptor and inhibits the hepatocyte mitochondrial gluconeogenic electron enzyme complex and increases the adenosine monophosphate (AMP). The AMP stimulates the AMP-activated protein kinase (AMPK), which reduces hepatic gluconeogenesis and increases the lactate production. Reproduced with permission from Pharmwiki, Tulane University Medical.

Evidence suggests that more intensive treatment of glycaemia in the newly diagnosed T2DM patients may reduce long-term cardiovascular diseases (CVD) rates.

The United Kingdom Prospective Diabetes Study (UKPDS) trial showed there was a 16% reduction in CVD events (combined fatal or nonfatal MI and sudden death) in the intensive glycaemic control arm that did not reach statistical significance, and there was no suggestion of benefit on other CVD outcomes (for example, stroke). However, after ten years of follow-up, those originally randomised to intensive glycemic control had significant long-term reductions in MI (15% with sulfonylurea or insulin as initial pharmacotherapy, 33% with metformin as initial pharmacotherapy) and in all-cause mortality (13% and 27%, respectively).[7] The pleiotropic effect of metformin needs to be confirmed with further randomised controlled trial.[8]

Common side effects include gastric distress (nausea, vomiting and diarrhoea). This can be overcome by using the sustained release Glucophage and escalating the dosages slowly over weeks.

Clinically relevant issues include patients undergoing contrast investigation who could potentially present with renal impairment, particularly those at high risk, including baseline renal impairment, liver, and heart failure. Patients with creatinine of 150 must not have metformin or prescribed metformin without proper assessment and consideration. It is contraindicated in those with lactic acidosis, ketoacidosis, dehydrated states, and severe organ failures.

## Thiazolidinediones (Glitazones)

This group of drugs caused quite a stir among the diabetic community after the discovery of increased heart failure deaths among those who received rosiglitazone.[9] This led to the withdrawal of the drug by the Food and Drug Authority in 2008. FDA has since then recommended that any future diabetic drugs must be tested for cardiovascular safety before approval. Only pioglitazone is currently on the market.

### Mechanism of Actions of Thiazolidinediones

The glitazones are insulin sensitizers. They bind on a nuclear receptor called the peroxisome proliferator-activated receptor gamma (PPARγ), which leads to the transcription of several genes involved in glucose and lipid metabolism. One of these transcriptions leads to the translation of GLUT-4 receptors, an insulin regulated glucose transporter found primarily on adipose tissue and striated muscles (skeletal & cardiac). GLUT-4 transporter vesicles fuse with the cell wall and allow glucose to enter the cells (**Figure 4.3**). This reduces insulin resistance and enhances its sensitivity leading to the reduction of hepatic gluconeogenesis, and, therefore, reduces blood glucose and HbA1c levels. Thus the glitazones do not stimulate insulin secretion but sensitize insulin secretion. They also reduce lipotoxicity by redistributing fat from muscle, liver, and pancreatic β cells to the subcutaneous depots.

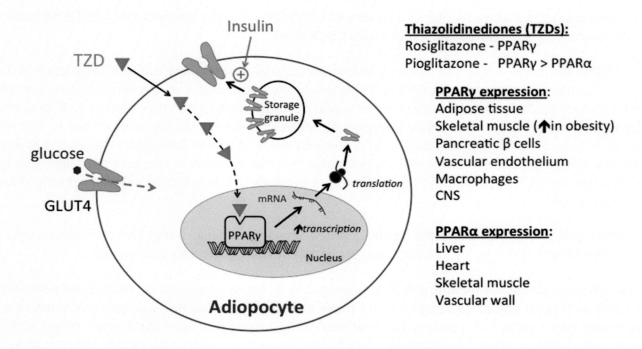

**Thiazolidinediones (TZDs):**
Rosiglitazone - PPARγ
Pioglitazone -  PPARγ > PPARα

**PPARγ expression:**
Adipose tissue
Skeletal muscle (↑in obesity)
Pancreatic β cells
Vascular endothelium
Macrophages
CNS

**PPARα expression:**
Liver
Heart
Skeletal muscle
Vascular wall

**Figure 4.3** Glitazones bind on PPARγ receptors in the nucleus, leading to translation of increased GLUT-4 receptors that increase glucose uptake. Reproduced with permission from PharmWiki, Tulane University School of Medicine.

The PROactive Study (**PRO**spective pioglit**A**zone **C**linical **T**rial **I**n macro**V**ascular **E**vents) indicates that patients with diabetes who were at high cardiovascular risk and were treated with pioglitazone showed improvement in insulin sensitivity, a reduction in the need for insulin, and improved cardiovascular outcome.[10]

The beneficial effects of the glitazones, notably pioglitazone, on cardiovascular function have also been linked to their pleiotropic effects, such as the reduction of the inflammatory markers and based on apparent differing effects on cardiovascular outcomes, pioglitazone is the preferred choice over rosiglitazone, particularly when low doses are administered.[11]

Side effects include weight gain, oedema, bone fractures, and cardiovascular risk.

---

- **Sulphonylureas are insulin secretagogues, have a glucose-independent hypoglycaemic effect and a three- to six-month hypoglycaemic 'wean-off effect', and potentially negate cardiovascular preconditioning.**

- **Pioglitazone is an insulin sensitiser and useful with pleiotropic effects on weight reduction and cardiovascular risk reduction and can be used in lean individuals who have insulin resistance.**

- **Metformin 'slows down' two key enzymes in hepatic gluconeogenesis (glucose 6-phosphate and phosphoenolpyruvate carboxykinase) without an apparent effect on lactate turnover for gluconeogenesis or increases in insulin secretion. Thus, fasting blood sugars are most affected. Metformin has pleiotropic effects that reduce CV outcomes through its 'metabolic memory'.**

---

**Newer Therapies**

## The Incretin Mimetics & Dipeptidyl Peptidase 4 Inhibitors
### Physiology of the Incretins

Incretins are two endogenous molecules produced from the enteroendocrine cells in the gut in response to presence of food in the stomach. Glucagon-like Peptide 1 (GLP-1) is secreted from the L-cells in the distal ileum and colon and glucose-dependent insulinotropic peptide (GIP) secreted from the K-cells in the jejunum (**Figure 4.4**).

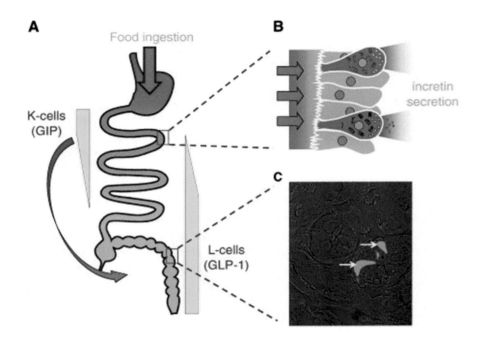

Figure 4.4 GLP-1 is produced from the L cell in the small intestine as proglucagon and converted into the active molecule the GLP-1. GIP is produced in the K cell of the proximal small intestine, jejunum, as ProGIP. Reproduced from Diakogiannaki, E., Gribble, F. M., & Reimann, F (2012). Nutrient detection by incretin hormone secreting cells. Physiology & behavior, 106(3), 387–393.

These molecules act on their receptors in the stomach by delaying gastric peristalsis, facilitate insulin secretion from the beta cells of the pancreas, reduce glycogenolysis in the liver by inhibiting release of glucagon, and cause early satiety by acting on their receptors in the satiety centre in the hypothalamus.[12] (**Figure 4.5**). They are broken down within two minutes by the enzyme diethyl peptide peptidase 4 (DPP-4).

The insulinotropic effect of GIP is completely lost in diabetes.[13] Therefore, GIP mimetics have not been developed as diabetes treatment, whilst GLP-1RAs and DPP-4 antagonists have been developed for diabetes treatment.[14]

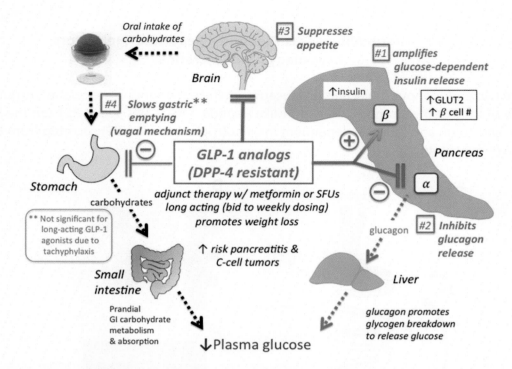

**Figure 4.5** (A) Release of the incretins from the intestine is stimulated by oral food intake. These increase insulin secretion, decrease glucagon secretion, and suppresses appetite. (B) The DPP-4 inhibitor group of drugs inhibit the DPP-4 enzymes breakdown of the incretins, and the GLP-1 agonists promotes serum levels of GLP1 peptide, thus, increase the incretin molecules concentration and their physiological effects. Reproduced with permission from PharmWiki, Tulane University School of Medicine.

### A. Glucagon-Like Peptide-1 Receptor Agonists (GLP-1RA) – Incretin Mimetic

GLP-1RAs are class of newer hypoglycaemic agents known as the incretin mimetic given as subcutaneous injections. They have been engineered to act like the biological GLP-1 but are resistant to breakdown by the degrading enzyme DPP-4. This allows sustained effects that ultimately lead to better glycaemic control (reduction of HBA1c by 1 to 1.5%) with good adjunctive effects of weight loss, no hypoglycaemia, drop in BP, lower lipids, and favourable CV profile. The GLP-1RAs have a glucose-dependent action unlike the sulphonylureas and, thus, have fewer hypoglycaemic effects.

They have an overall effect on the reduction of both the fasting plasma glucose (FPG), and the postprandial glucose (PPG) but predominantly the PPG. They are used in combination treatment with insulins, particularly the basal insulin to achieve optimal glycaemic controls. This strategy is based on several caveats:

- Basal insulins control the FPG, and the GLP-1RAs control the PPG.
- GLP-1RAs antagonise the hypoglycaemic and weight gain effects of insulins.
- Use of GLP-1RAs allows for reduction in the insulin dosage.

These principles have been shown in studies to offer better glycaemic control and accord other beneficial CV effects in controlling the conventional CV risk factors.

The GLP-1RAs as a class have transient gastric intolerant effect characterised by nausea, vomiting, and diarrhoea that could last less than two weeks. The long-acting GLP1-RAs, however, have reduced gastrointestinal side effects.

The ADA/EASD have stated that current evidence lacks concrete association between the GLP-1RA, pancreatitis and pancreatic cancer. ADA/EASD however, recommends the cautious use of the GLP-1RA in patients at risk of these conditions.

*Types of GLP-1RAs*

There are two categories of GLP-1RAs currently being used in clinical practice based on their duration of actions. They are all injectables with one oral preparation (semaglutide

- *Short-acting—used twice daily*
  - Lixistenatide 10mcg daily for two weeks and escalate to 20mcg daily thereafter
  - Exenatide (immediate release) Initially, 5 micrograms twice daily for at least one month and then increased if necessary up to 10 micrograms twice daily; doses to be taken within one hour before two main meals (at least six hours apart)
  - Liraglutide 0.6mcg daily and increase dose after 1 week to 1.2mcg and further 1.8mcg if necessary

- *Long-acting—used daily*
  - Liraglutide- 0.6mg daily and increase dose by 0.6mg weekly until 3mg daily as maintenance
  - Albiglutide-30 mg subcutaneously once a week. If glycemic response is inadequate, may increase to 50 mg subcutaneously once a week. Maintenance dose: 30 or 50 mg subcutaneously once a week
  - Exenatide—modified release, 2 micrograms once weekly
  - Dulaglutide - 0.75 mg weekly; increase to 1.5 mg or up to 4 mg after 6 to 8 weeks.
  - Semaglutide- 0.25 mg the first four weeks; 0.5 mg thereafter and to 1mg weekly.
  - Semaglutide- 3mg po daily for 1 month followed by 7mg for another month and escalated to 14mg daily

### Two Classes of GLP-1RAs

1. Short-acting GLP-1RAs
2. Long-acting GLP1RAs

**GLP-1RAs are insulin secretagogues with 'glucose-dependent' action (no hypoglycaemia) and predominantly control the PPG. They offer variable strategies in glycaemic control with insulin and have positive effects on cardiovascular outcomes.**

### B. Dipeptidyl Peptidase-4 Inhibitors (DPP-4 Inhibitors): Gliptins

The gliptins inhibit the DPP-4 enzyme from breaking down the GLP-1 and GLP. This promotes prolonged physiological effects of these hormones.

They have effects on both the FPG and the PPG but predominantly on PPG and have a modest effect on glycaemic control with reduction of HBA1c by 0.5 to 1%. They do not have hypoglycaemic effects (glucose-dependent insulin secretion) and are weight neutral. In addition, they reduce blood pressure by 2.5 mmHg.[15] However, there is a trend of increased heart failure admission among diabetic patients at high risk of heart failure without increase in ischemic events.[16] The most common side effects include headaches and upper respiratory tract infections.

They can be used as a first- and/or second-line antidiabetic treatment in association with others when glycaemic control is not achieved and/or use of other medications are contraindicated.[17]

There are five gliptin drugs currently on the market:

- Alogliptin
- Sitagliptin
- Saxagliptin
- Linagliptin
- Vildagliptin

Fixed-dose combinations are:

- Kazano = alogliptin/metformin (12.5 mg / 50 or 1000 mg) bd daily
- Janumet = sitagliptin/metformin has various strengths (50 mg/500 mg, 50 mg/1,000 mg, 100 mg/1,000 mg) bd daily
- Galvus Met = vildagliptin/metformin (50 mg/500 mg or 50 mg/1,000mg)

---

**The gliptins have minimal glycaemic control with a tendency towards precipitating heart failure episodes in high-risk patients.**

---

### C. The Sodium-Glucose Transporters Inhibitors (SGLT2 Receptor Antagonists)

*Role of Kidneys in Glucose Metabolism*

The kidneys produce 20% of fasting glucose and contribute to 100% reabsorption of the filtered glucose in the urine of non-diabetic people through the sodium-glucose co-transporters in the kidney tubules. The SGLT2 and the SGLT1 transporters located in the proximal tubules are responsible for the reabsorption of virtually 100% of the filtered glucose load.

On average, the kidneys filter about 180 grams of glucose every day. In normal glucose-tolerant individuals, the kidneys reabsorb all the filtered glucose, and virtually no glucose appears in the urine. The SGLT2 transporters, which are in the first portion of the proximal tubule, reabsorb 90% of the filtered glucose load while the SGLT1 transporters, located in the more distal S2-S3 segments of the proximal tubule, reabsorb the remaining 10% of the filtered glucose load.[18]

---

**Kidneys contribute 20% of fasting glucose through gluconeogenesis and glucose reabsorption, the liver contributes 70%, and muscles and adipose tissues contribute 10%.**

---

*SGLT2 Receptor Antagonists*

SGLT2 inhibitors are called 'new therapy,' compared with the traditional diabetic drugs, though, they have been in use for over a decade now.

There are four SGLT2-receptor antagonists on the market and used daily:

- Empagliflozin—10 mg daily increased to 25 mg daily if tolerated
- Dapagliflozin—5 mg, 10 mg
- Canagliflozin—100 mg daily and can be increased to 300 mg daily if tolerated
- Ertugliflozin—5mg daily and increased to 15 mg once daily if necessary

They can be used as monotherapy and/or dual therapy in situations where metformin is contraindicated or glycaemic control is not achieved with other treatment, such as insulin.

Studies have shown that the SGLT2 receptors are greatly increased in patients with T2DM. This leads to an increase in glucose reabsorption and a rise in the threshold of glucose excretion in the urine, which inadvertently raises the plasma glucose levels.

The use of the SGLT2 antagonists has been shown to reduce the threshold of glucose excretion, improve insulin secretion by negating the glucotoxic effects on the Beta cell function, and reduces HBA1c by 0.7 to 1%.

Other pleiotropic effects include weight loss due to the osmotic diuretic effect, reduction in blood pressure, and reduction in heart failure deaths and events among both diabetic and non-diabetic patients.[19] These have led to the use of the SGLT2 antagonists in the treatment of both the diabetic and the non-diabetic patients with heart failure. [20]

Patients with diabetes frequently have diabetic nephropathy. The use of the SGLT2 antagonists is also beneficial to those with CKD. There would be an initial dip of 3-6ml/min in eGFR in the first 4-6 weeks but there will be regain in some function in approximately 12 weeks. [21] The "permissive hypercreatininemia" is considered a bona fide marker of long-term benefit. However, it is not recommended for those with an eGFR ≤20ml/min.

SGLT2 antagonists have a class effect of causing euglycaemic diabetic ketoacidosis. Patients must be informed of effects of ketoacidosis so that they seek medical attention when they develop rapid weight loss, sweet smelling breath, fast breathing, abdominal pain, nausea, and vomiting.

The SGLT2 antagonists additionally cause recurrent urinary tract infection and balanitis in uncircumcised males. Treatment of the UTI remains the same as those who are not diabetic. Fournier's gangrene is a dangerous skin infection that can happen in patients treated with SGLT2-receptor antagonists. The drugs must be stopped, patients admitted, antibiotics started, and surgical debridement considered.

### Effects of SGLT2 Antagonists ·

- Inhibition of glucose reabsorption in proximal tubule, thereby increasing glucose excretion through urine
- Weight loss due to osmotic diuretic effect
- Reduction of blood pressure
- Reduction of heart failure admissions and deaths in both diabetic and non-diabetic patients
- Euglycemic ketoacidosis
- Risk of UTI and, in uncircumcised males, balanitis

*Mechanism of Action of SGLT-2 Antagonists*

The SGLT2 receptors in the proximal renal tubules facilitate 90% of glucose absorption from the kidney. The SGLT-2 antagonists are a class of diabetic drugs that bind on these sodium-glucose transporters 2 and block reabsorption of filtered glucose from the glomeruli. This allows excess glucose to be secreted by the kidneys through urine, as shown in **Figure 4.6**. They have an insulin-independent mechanism without causing hypoglycaemia

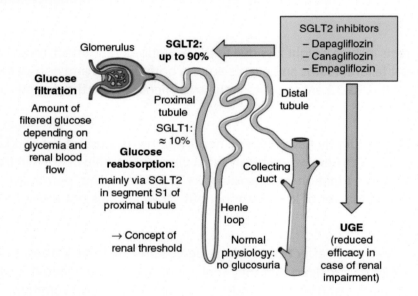

**Figure 4.6** SGLT2 inhibitors act on SGLT2 receptors in proximal renal convoluted tubules and reduce renal glucosuric threshold, thereby increasing renal glucose excretion. Reproduced with permission from Scheen A. J. Evaluating SGLT2 inhibitors for type 2 diabetes: pharmacokinetic and toxicological considerations. *Expert opinion on drug metabolism & toxicology, 10*(5), 647–663.

**SGLT2 antagonists have insulin-independent action through glucose secretion. They have pleiotropic effects—good glycaemic control, weight loss, and reduced heart failure—but can cause euglycemic ketosis, urinary tract infection, and a tendency towards limb amputation.**

**D. Insulin**

Insulin is covered in chapter 5. The discussion in this section is on new insulins manufactured in the 1990s. Modern insulin analogues were produced in the 1990s by the biochemical alteration of the insulin molecule. These insulins comparatively provide better glycaemic control, less hypoglycaemia, and less weight gain than its older human insulin counterparts.

*Modern Ultra Short-Acting Insulin Analogues*

- Aspart
- Lispro
- Glulisine

*First-Generation Long-Acting Basal Insulins*

- Detemir
- Glargine

*Second-Generation Basal Insulin*

- Degludec (less variability, less hypoglycaemia/nocturnal hypoglycaemia, can be co-formulated unlike the first generation)

*Co-Formulated Degludec*

- Degludec/Aspart
- Degludec/Liraglutide

## Optimisation of Glycaemic Control

The primary objective of diabetes treatment is to achieve optimal glycaemic control without causing hypoglycaemia or untoward side effects of diabetic drugs. The surrogate for glycaemic control is HBA1c level, and physicians attempt several cocktails of diabetic medications regimens as recommended in the 2015 ADA/EASD guidelines to reach their pre-treatment targets based on the individual needs and values in a so-called patient-centred, individualised approach.

There are several steps involved in the optimisation of glycaemic control:

- Diagnosis of the type of diabetes
- Assessment of clinical status and characteristics of the patient
- Setting a target HBA1c level and targets of other conventional cardiovascular risk factors
- Treatment initiation with a treatment regimen
- Review three months with HBA1c (Not with T1DM)
- Optimise treatment to achieve target

The target for optimisation is underpinned by several factors—age of the patient, duration of diabetes, presence or absence of complications, health service delivery capacities, and the motivation of the patients.

The ADA and the EASD have released a consensus guideline on personalised care of the diabetic patients using a stepwise treatment escalation algorithm approach to pharmacotherapy.

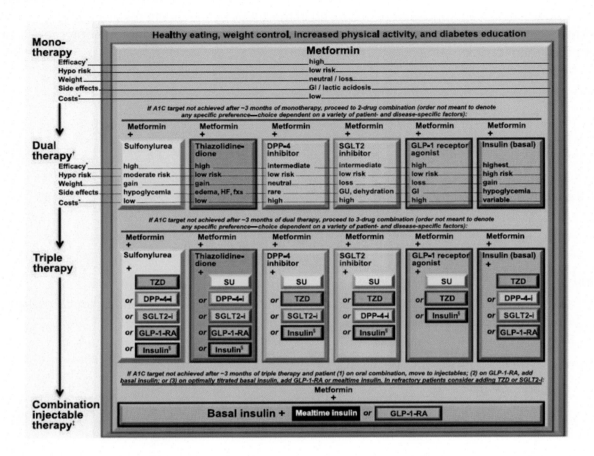

**Figure 4.7** Diabetes treatment algorithm. Reproduced from Inzucchi et.al., 'Management of Hyperglycaemia in Type 2 Diabetes: A Patient-Centred Approach', *Diabetes Care*, 35/6 (2012), 1,364–79.

## Key Messages:

- **Management of diabetes is based on the three pillars of dieting, exercise, and pharmacotherapy.**
- **Premedical assessment precedes any exercise prescriptions.**
- **Metformin remains the first-choice pharmacotherapy in T2DM and escalation with other drugs in a personalized approach. Insulin can be used as monotherapy or dual therapy in selective cases.**
- **The SGLT2 antagonists are novel in reducing heart failure morbidity and mortality in both the diabetic and the non-diabetic heart failure patients.**

## References:

1    Colberg, S. R., Sigal, R. J., Fernhall, B., et.al., American College of Sports Medicine, & American Diabetes Association (2010). Exercise and type 2 diabetes: the American College of Sports Medicine and the American Diabetes Association: joint position statement. *Diabetes care*, 33(12), e147–e167. https://doi.org/10.2337/dc10-9990.

2    Ryerson, B., Tierney, E. F., Thompson, T. J., Engelgau,et.al., (2003). Excess physical limitations among adults with diabetes in the U.S. population, 1997-1999. *Diabetes care*, 26(1), 206–210. https://doi.org/10.2337/diacare.26.1.206.

3   Marwick, T. H., Hordern, M. D., Miller, T., Chyun, et.al., & Council on Clinical Cardiology, American Heart Association Exercise, Cardiac Rehabilitation, and Prevention Committee, Council on Cardiovascular Disease in the Young, Council on Cardiovascular Nursing, Council on Nutrition, Physical Activity, and Metabolism, & Interdisciplinary Council on Quality of Care and Outcomes Research (2009). Exercise training for type 2 diabetes mellitus: impact on cardiovascular risk: a scientific statement from the American Heart Association. *Circulation*, *119*(25), 3244–3262. https://doi.org/10.1161/CIRCULATIONAHA.109.192521.

4   Ashcroft F. M. (1996). Mechanisms of the glycaemic effects of sulfonylureas. *Hormone and metabolic 28*(9), 456–463. https://doi.org/10.1055/s-2007-979837

5   Tomai, F., Crea, F., Chiariello, L., & Gioffrè, P. A. (1999). Ischemic preconditioning in humans: models, mediators, and clinical relevance. *Circulation*, *100*(5), 559–563. https://doi.org/10.1161/01.cir.100.5.559 .

6   Kirpichnikov, D., McFarlane, S. I., & Sowers, J. R. (2002). Metformin: an update. *Annals of internal medicine, 137*(1), 25–33. https://doi.org/10.7326/0003-4819-137-1-200207020-00009

7   Holman, R. R., Paul, S. K., Bethel, M. A.,et.al.,(2008). 10-year follow-up of intensive glucose control in type 2 diabetes. *The New England journal of medicine, 359*(15), 1577–1589. https://doi.org/10.1056/NEJMoa0806470.

8   Bromage, D. I., & Yellon, D. M. (2015). The pleiotropic effects of metformin: time for prospective studies. *Cardiovascular diabetology, 14*, 109. https://doi.org/10.1186/s12933-015-0273-5.

9   Nissen, S. E., & Wolski, K. (2007). Effect of rosiglitazone on the risk of myocardial infarction and death from cardiovascular causes. *The New England journal of medicine, 356*(24), 2457–2471. https://doi.org/10.1056/NEJMoa072761.

10  Dormandy, J. A., Charbonnel, B., Eckland, D. J., et.,al., PROactive Investigators (2005). Secondary prevention of macrovascular events in patients with type 2 diabetes in the PROactive Study (PROspective pioglitAzone Clinical Trial In macroVascular Events): a randomised controlled trial. *Lancet (London, England), 366*(9493), 1279–1289. https://doi.org/10.1016/S0140-6736(05)67528-9

11  Defronzo, R. A., Mehta, R. J., & Schnure, J. J. (2013). Pleiotropic effects of thiazolidinediones: implications for the treatment of patients with type 2 diabetes mellitus. *Hospital practice (1995), 41*(2), 132–147. https://doi.org/10.3810/hp.2013.04.1062.

12  Diabetes UK, Incretins Mimetics/GLP-1. https://www.diabetes.org.uk/incretin-mimetics.

13  Aaboe, K., Krarup, T., Madsbad, S., & Holst, J. J. (2008). GLP-1: physiological effects and potential therapeutic applications. *Diabetes, obesity & metabolism, 10*(11), 994–1003. https://doi.org/10.1111/j.1463-1326.2008.00853.

14  Girard J. (2008). The incretins: from the concept to their use in the treatment of type 2 diabetes. Part A: incretins: concept and physiological functions. *Diabetes & metabolism, 34*(6 Pt 1), 550–559. https://doi.org/10.1016/j.diabet.2008.09.001

15  Blonde, L., & Russell-Jones, D. (2009). The safety and efficacy of liraglutide with or without oral antidiabetic drug therapy in type 2 diabetes: an overview of the LEAD 1-5 studies. *Diabetes, obesity & metabolism, 11 Suppl 3*, 26–34. https://doi.org/10.1111/j.1463-1326.2009.01075.x

16  Scirica, B. M., Bhatt, D. L., Braunwald, E., et.al., & SAVOR-TIMI 53 Steering Committee and Investigators (2013). Saxagliptin and cardiovascular outcomes in patients with type 2 diabetes mellitus. *The New England journal of medicine, 369*(14), 1317–1326. https://doi.org/10.1056/NEJMoa1307684.

17  Inzucchi, S. E., Bergenstal, R. M., Buse, J. B.,et.,al., American Diabetes Association (ADA), & European Association for the Study of Diabetes (EASD) (2012). Management of hyperglycemia in type 2 diabetes: a patient-centered approach: position statement of the American Diabetes Association (ADA) and the European Association for the Study of Diabetes (EASD). *Diabetes care, 35*(6), 1364–1379. https://doi.org/10.2337/dc12-0413

18  Wilding J. P. (2014). The role of the kidneys in glucose homeostasis in type 2 diabetes: clinical implications and therapeutic significance through sodium glucose co-transporter 2 inhibitors. *Metabolism: clinical and experimental, 63*(10), 1228–1237. https://doi.org/10.1016/j.metabol.2014.06.018

19  McMurray, J., Solomon, S. D., Inzucchi, S. E., et., DAPA-HF Trial Committees and Investigators (2019). Dapagliflozin in Patients with Heart Failure and Reduced Ejection Fraction. *The New England journal of medicine, 381*(21), 1995–2008. https://doi.org/10.1056/NEJMoa1911303

20  Ponikowski, P., Voors, A. A., Anker, S. D., et.al., & ESC Scientific Document Group (2016). 2016 ESC Guidelines for the diagnosis and treatment of acute and chronic heart failure: The Task Force for the diagnosis and treatment of acute and chronic heart failure of the European Society of Cardiology (ESC)Developed with the special contribution of the Heart Failure Association (HFA) of the ESC. *European heart journal, 37*(27), 2129–2200. https://doi.org/10.1093/eurheartj/ehw128

21  Meraz-Muñoz, A. Y., Weinstein, J., & Wald, R. (2021). eGFR Decline after SGLT2 Inhibitor Initiation: The Tortoise and the Hare Reimagined. *Kidney360, 2*(6), 1042–1047. https://doi.org/10.34067/KID.0001172021

# CHAPTER 5
# Insulin Management

Diabetes should only be a word not a life sentence.
**Author Unknown**

## History of Insulin

The discovery of insulin in 1921 and its subsequent purification, modification, and DNA biosynthetic engineering have changed the perception of diabetes as a disease with a death sentence to a chronic disease that is manageable. Its development over the following five decades have been progressive, from short-acting immunogenic animal extracts to purified human insulin engineered into bacteria and yeast for mass production for commercial purposes. **Table 5.1** gives a timeline of this medical breakthrough.[1],[2]

---

### History of Insulin Development

**1921.** Insulin discovery
- Extracts from cow and pigs were used with short action and were very immunogenic, as they contained other peptides that stimulated antibody production.

**1930s.** Modifications of insulin pharmacokinetic properties
- Compounds such as zinc and protamine were added to delay absorption and prolong insulin activity.
- Intermediate insulins were, thus, produced.

**1972.** Insulin purification
- Chromatography was used to separate insulin from other pancreatic peptides to produce pure insulin molecules.

**1980.** Human insulin production
- Human insulin gene was engineered into bacteria and yeast to produce large amounts of insulin for commercial purposes.

**1990.** Analogue insulin production
- Analogue insulins were made by small changes in the amino acid chain to confer specific pharmacokinetic properties deemed desirable.
- Short-acting analogues (aspart, lispro, glusine) and first-generation long-acting (determir and glargine) were produced.

**2000.** Production of second-generation analogue and fixed-dose combination
- Second-generation long-acting basal insulin analogues (degludec) and fixed dose combinations (degludec/liraglutide) were developed.

---

Table 5.1 Insulin developmental timeline.

**The evolution of insulin involved refining short-acting, highly immunogenic biological insulin to intermediate and long-acting non-immunogenic synthetic insulin (human insulin) with mass production using recombinant DNA technology.**

## Physiology of Insulin Production and Secretion

Insulin is a polypeptide hormone of two chains. The alpha chain has twenty-one amino acids, and the beta chain has thirty amino acids connected by two disulphide bridges. It is synthesised in the ßeta cells of the islets of Langerhans of the pancreas and is initially formed as pre-proinsulin. Its beta and alpha chains of amino acids are connected by C-peptide with the NH3 signal sequence attached to the terminal of the beta chain. The process of proteolysis results in the removal of the NH3 signal sequence to proinsulin. Further removal of the C-peptide results in the functional insulin molecule.[3] (**Figure 5.1**)

**Formation of Insulin**

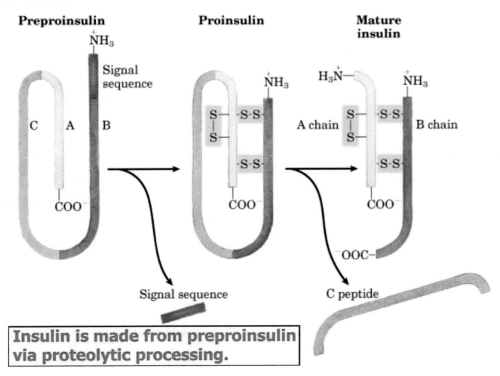

**Figure 5.1** Procession of preproinsulin to active insulin via enzymatic proteolysis in the ßeta cells of the islets of Langerhans cells of the pancreas. S-S = Sulphide bond. Reproduced from Thompson A, Kanamarlapudi V (2013) Type 2 Diabetes Mellitus and Glucagon Like Peptide-1 Receptor Signalling. Clin Exp Pharmacol 3: 138.

**Insulin production in the ßeta cells is by the translation of insulin mRNA into preproinsulin in the endoplasmic reticulum, followed by endopeptidase cleavage of NH3 signal sequence to proinsulin. Proinsulin is further cleaved to insulin and exported to the Golgi bodies for packaging and stored in granules ready for release.**

## Glucose Mediated Insulin Secretion

Insulin is secreted from the ßeta cells of the islets of Langerhans. This process of secretion is mediated by the uptake of glucose via the GLUT2 receptors located along the borders of the ßeta cells. Glucose enters the ßeta cells and undergoes glycolysis. The AcetylCoA produced from this glycolysis enters the Krebs Cycle in the mitochondria to produce more ATPs for the cells' intrinsic metabolic needs. The ATP produced from this process drives the exudation of K+ causing depolarisation of the cell nucleus. Calcium in the plasma fluid enters the ßeta cell nucleus via the voltage gated L- type $Ca^{2}+$ channels and repolarises the nucleus, leading to secretion of insulin. [4] (**Figure 5.2**)

Secretion of insulin in the physiological state is *biphasic*. Basal insulin is continuously secreted at a rate of 0.5 to 1 units/kg to maintain the fasting glucose produced from the processes of gluconeogenesis from the liver/kidneys and glycogenolysis from adipose tissue. The second phase of insulin secretion is after eating to control the postprandial glucose excursion. The principle of insulin therapy is to simulate the natural biphasic insulin secretion as much as possible.

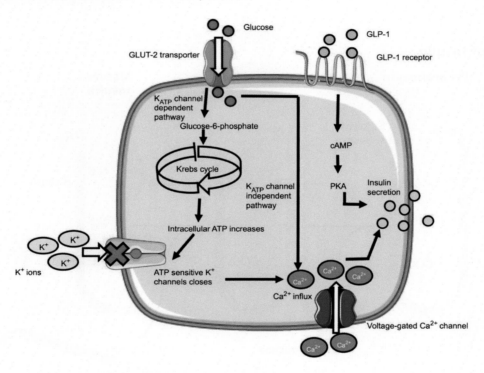

**Figure 5.2** Mechanism of insulin secretion from ß-cells in response to glucose (left) and GLP-1 (right). Adapted from *Ojha A et al.* Current perspective on the role of insulin and glucagon in the pathogenesis and treatment of type 2 diabetes mellitus. *Clinical Pharmacology: Advances and Applications 2019:11 57-65'* Originally published by and used with permission from Dove Medical Press Ltd.

---

**The release of insulin is initiated by entry of glucose through GLUT2 receptors on the ßeta cells, followed by the process of glycolysis in the cytoplasm of the ßeta cell.**

**AcetylCoA produced enters Krebs cycle in mitochondria to generate more ATPs that exude K+ from the ßeta cell cytoplasm. Entry of Ca2+ through voltage-gated calcium channels depolarises the plasma of the ßeta cell, leading to degranulation of the insulin granules into the plasma.**

---

# Classification of Insulins

Insulins are essentially classified based on their duration of actions. These include:

1. *Rapid-acting insulin*. Humalog, Novolog, or Apidra. This insulin is taken before or immediately after eating to counteract the rise in blood sugar from the food. It begins to work in fifteen to thirty minutes, peaks in one and a half to two hours, and lasts four hours.
2. *Short-acting insulin*. Regular or R insulins, examples include Actrapid and NovoRapid. This group begins to work within an hour but stops working sooner than intermediate or long-acting insulins, peaks in two to four hours, and lasts for six to eight hours.
3. *Intermediate-acting insulin*. NPH (N) and Lente (L) peak in six to twelve hours and last eighteen to twenty-six hours
4. *Long-acting insulin*. Lantus and Levemir begin to act in six to eight hours, peak in fourteen to twenty-four hours, and last twenty-eight to thirty-six hours. Degludec (Tresiba) peaks in eight to twelve hours, is effective up to forty-two hours, and has onset of action from two to four hours.
5. *Pre-mixed insulin*. These groups have a short-acting and an intermediate-acting and or long-acting basal insulin. Examples include Mixtard (Actrapid + NPH), NovoMix (Aspart + NPH), Humulin M3, Homolog Mix 25 75/25, and Homolog Mix 50 50/50.

| Administered at mealtimes (just before or after meals) | Administered 30mins before meal or immediately after if unpredictable | Administered once or twice a day (Not dependent on mealtimes) |
|---|---|---|
| Rapid Acting Insulins | Short Acting Insulins<br>Biphasic or Pre-mixed Insulins | Basal or Background Insulin |
| Insulin Glulisine (Apidra)<br>Insulin Lispro (Humalog)<br>Insulin Aspart (Novorapid)<br>Hypurine Bovine Neutral<br>Hypurin Porcine Neutral | Human Actrapid<br>Human S<br>Insuman Rapid<br>Humalog Mix 25<br>Humalog Mix 50<br>Humulin M3<br>Insuman Comb 25<br>Insuman Comb 50<br>Novomix 30 | Humulin I<br>Human Insulatard<br>Hypurin Bovine Isophane<br>Hypurin Porcine Isophane<br>Insulin Glargine (Lantus)<br>Insulin Determir (Levemir)<br>Insuman Basal |

Table 5.2: Types of Insulin based on their duration of action

# Indications for Initiation of Insulin Therapy in Diabetes

### Initiation of Insulin in Type 1 Diabetes

Patients with T1DM automatically qualify for insulin therapy, although some hybrid forms of diabetes such as LADA and MODY would have a delayed initiation.

### Initiation of Insulin in Type 2 Diabetes Mellitus

It is difficult to have a generic guideline on insulin initiation for type 2 diabetes. However, a few caveats must be taken into consideration when planning insulin therapy:

• Clinical and biochemical indications for initiation of insulin

- Patient's clinical profile (duration of diabetes, presence of complications, comorbidities, available support services and treatment intensities)
- Patient's understanding of insulin therapy, education, support in decision making and allaying misconceptions and fears of insulin therapy (decisions must always be made in the patient's best interest)
- Overcoming physicians own inertia

## Essential Indications

- Signs of glucotoxicity (polyuria, polyphagia, polydipsia, and weight loss)
- Random blood glucose of ≥16 mmol/L
- HBA1c 9%
- Uncontrolled blood glucose whilst on dual and or triple therapy
- Ketoacidosis
- Diabetic patients with acute coronary syndromes

## Early or Late Insulinisation

The initiation of insulin as the 'last line of defence' was the traditional treatment approach taken by the medical community over decades for the treatment of T2DM. This practice involves a step-up protocol, where insulin is added as either dual or triple therapy when the glycaemic control is not achieved with other agents on optimal their dosages. This is evident in the recent ADA/EASD guideline criteria for initiation of insulin, where it is stated, 'Insulin can be initiated in dual or triple therapy with metformin/SU/GLP-1Ras.'[4]

Recent evidence suggests that early initiation of insulin preserves ßeta cell function and delays chronic complications. [5] In addition, the late initiation and treatment with insulin has been shown to have negative effects on those with advanced diabetes (ACCORD Study).[6] Clinical inertia (physician and patient) also plays a significant role in promulgating the development of complications. These have led to the promotion of early insulin therapy (Insulinisation). Therefore the early insulinisation in T2DM with certain clinical profiles is observed to confer benefits with optimal glycaemic control and the reduction of complications. These profile include:

- Severely hyperglycaemic patients
- Those with a more pronounced increase in FPG than in PPG
- Leaner patients because they are less likely to gain weight and are more likely to be insulin deficient
- Obese patients who take insulin in combination with a GLP-1 receptor agonist
- Patients taking a GLP-1 receptor agonist whose FPG remains high
- Patients with a positive attitude about insulin therapy who are more likely to achieve higher remission rates

The decision to initiate insulin therapy early or later is to be made by the patients, with provision of sufficient information and support from the healthcare practitioner. Understanding the status of the diabetes, the clinical profile, and the preferences of the patient, along with adequate discussions of all the risks and benefits, will lead towards a mutually agreed plan of action.

The next stage is for both parties to agree on a personalised treatment target and individualisation of the treatment approach which can be either standard or intensive treatment strategy.

## Intensive versus Standard Insulin Treatment Approach

The intensive approach is appropriate for the newly diagnosed with no complications. Young patients with diabetes less than 5 years duration, and those able to monitor their blood glucose. The Diabetes Control and Complication Trial (DCCT) has shown that intensive insulin treatment led to the reduction in chronic microvascular complication. [7]

The less intensive glycaemic control can be accorded to the elderly patients, those with established diabetic complications, and brittle diabetes, as the ACCORD Study has shown that intensive treatment leads to high mortality.

The UKPDS and Kumamoto Trials in T2DM showed microvascular complications were significantly reduced in the intensive insulin arm. [8,9] Patients continued to have reduced chronic complications despite being off the intensive protocol after many years. [10]

The approach to management of hyperglycaemia is now personalised based on these dichotomised results of insulin management approaches which is based on the patient profile as shown in **Figure 5.3**.

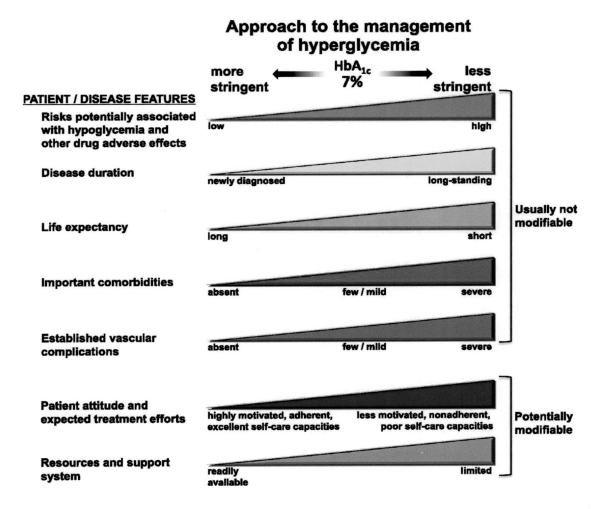

**Figure 5.3** Customised glycaemic control approach according to the profile of patient. Reproduced from Silvio E. Inzucchi, et al., 'Management of Hyperglycaemia in Type 2 Diabetes, 2015: A Patient-Centered Approach: Update to a Position Statement of the American Diabetes Association and the European Association for the Study of Diabetes', *Diabetes Care* 38/1 (Jan 2015), 140–49

**Insulin initiation can be either early or late and can be either intensive or standard depending on patients' clinical and biochemical profiles, their understanding of the treatment approaches, and their wishes.**

## Insulin Dosages

It is difficult to have a fixed-dose regimen of insulin for every diabetic patient. However, some basic principles in insulin prescription must be understood to initiate and monitor the therapy.

- Insulin is secreted in a bimodal fashion by a normal functioning pancreas to control the fasting and the postprandial glucose (**Figure 5.4**). Insulin therapy is essentially to replicate and/or enhance the biological phases of secretions.
- Basal insulin is estimated to be 0.5 to 1unit per kg. For example, an eighty-kilogram man will have a basal insulin requirement of 40 to 80 units of insulin daily.
- Postprandial insulin can be a short-acting insulin prescribed in a low-escalating dose, based on the postprandial glycaemic excursions.
- Those patients who undergo education on carbohydrate count and on CSII can estimate variable insulin doses depending on their carbohydrate intake count.

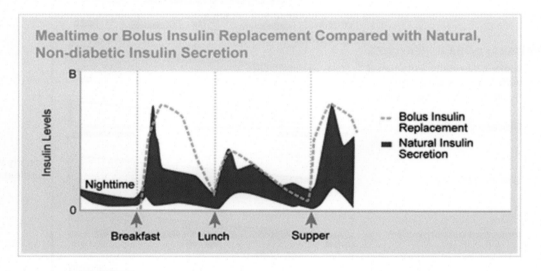

**Figure 5.4** Basal (natural) insulin secretion is continuous and surges after meals (postprandial). Exogenous basal insulin is given to augment the endogenous basal insulin secretion to control the fasting glucose. Exogenous bolus insulin is given to augment endogenous postprandial insulin secretion to control postprandial glucose excursions . Reproduced with permission from Jacobs, M. A, et.al. (1997). Metabolic efficacy of preprandial administration of Lys(B28), Pro(B29) human insulin analog in IDDM patients. A comparison with human regular insulin during a three-meal test period. *Diabetes care, 20*(8), 1279–1286.

**Exogenous insulin is prescribed to mimic the biphasic physiological secretions, quite often using the basal bolus principle:**

- **Basal insulin – insulin secreted by pancreas**
- **Bolus insulin – insulin secreted by pancreas after meals**

**Insulin Regimens**

There are six different insulin regimens that can be delivered to diabetic patients based on several factors—patient profile, availability, costs, and the insulin profile.

- **Once Daily Basal Insulin**

  In this regimen, either the long-acting insulin (glargine, determir, and degludec) or the intermediate-acting insulin, such as isophane insulin (Humulin I or Insulatard) are used

- **Basal-Plus Regimen**

  This regimen involves a basal insulin plus a short acting or ultrashort acting insulin postprandial as and when required to control the PPG surge. It attempts to simulate the physiological bimodal insulin secretion. Compared with a basal insulin regimen, this regimen is better and effective in reducing HBA1c levels.[11] Insulin degludec co-formulated with insulin aspart has been shown to improved glycaemic control with less hypoglycaemic episodes and could be used for such purpose.

- **Premix Insulin**

  Is a mixture of intermediate and rapid-acting insulins in one mixture given twice daily as a simple regimen for those needing a simple regimen like the elderly, visually impaired and or in insulin naive patients starting treatment. This regimen is disadvantaged by poor glycaemic control, increased hypoglycaemia and reduces patients flexibility in timing of their meals. It is rigid and must be taken with fixed meal schedules. It's convenient for patients and suitable for resource limited settings and is quite popular in many developing countries.

- **Basal Bolus Insulin**

  This regimen attempts to simulate the physiological insulin secretion with a basal insulin and a short acting insulin as prandial insulin after meals to control the post prandial glucose surge. The ultra short acting and or short acting insulins are used as bolus insulin after meals. (**Figure 5.4**).

- **Basal Insulin/Incretin Combinations**

  There are two patterns of this strategy: GLP1RAs on insulin or Insulin on GLP1RAs. Collectively, these combinations have improved glycaemic control, reduced hypoglycaemia and weight gain seen among insulin treated patients The GLP-1RA are now used with the basal insulins to complement each other and negate some of insulin's untoward effects such as the weight gain, hypoglycemia. The complimentary effect of the GLP-1RA is significant on the postprandial glycaemic control allowing for a dose reduction of insulin.

- **Continuous Subcutaneous Insulin Infusion (CSII)**

  Patients whose blood sugar fluctuates wildly despite multiple daily insulin injection regimen therapy qualify for CSII. Currently, many young and middle-aged people are the users of CSII. This is currently prescribed by a qualified diabetic physician and/or endocrinologist in the United Kingdom. The machine costs between £2,000 - £3000 depending on the supplier. (**Figure 5.5**)

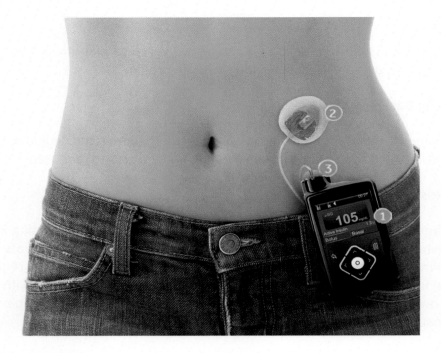

**Figure 5.5** An insulin pump that is attached to the skin. Insulin dosage instructions are added to the pump, which pumps controlled insulin into the subcutaneous tissue through a catheter embedded through the skin. Reproduced with permission from Medtronic.

### *Insulin Regimens*

- Basal insulin
- Basal Plus
- Basal Bolus
- Premix
- Basal plus incretin combination
- Continuous subcutaneous insulin infusion

## Key Messages

- **Insulin has changed the fate of diabetes; once a fatal disease, it is now a chronic manageable disease.**
- **Insulin is prescribed in various regimens to simulate the physiological biphasic secretion.**
- **Early insulinisation has shown to remit and control blood glucose and retard chronic complications.**
- **Insulin can be prescribed as monotherapy, dual, and/or triple therapy.**
- **Prescription of insulin is according to indications and customised to the patient profile.**

# References:

1  History of Insulin. Diabetes UK. https://www.diabetes.co.uk/insulin/history-of-insulin.html.

2  P. J. Watkins, S. A. Amiel, S. L. Howell, and E. Turner *Diabetes and its management*, 6th edn (Carlton, Victoria, Australia: Blackwell Publishing).

3  Vasiljević, J., Torkko, J. M., Knoch, K. P., & Solimena, M. (2020). The making of insulin in health and disease. *Diabetologia*, *63*(10), 1981–1989. https://doi.org/10.1007/s00125-020-05192-7J.

4  Inzucchi, S. E., Bergenstal, R. M., Buse, J. B, et. al., (2012). Management of hyperglycaemia in type 2 diabetes: a patient-centered approach. Position statement of the American Diabetes Association (ADA) and the European Association for the Study of Diabetes (EASD). *Diabetologia*, *55*(6), 1577–1596. https://doi.org/10.1007/s00125-012-2534-0

5  Pennartz, C., Schenker, N., Menge, B. A., et. al., 2011). Chronic reduction of fasting glycemia with insulin glargine improves first- and second-phase insulin secretion in patients with type 2 diabetes. *Diabetes care*, *34*(9), 2048–2053. https://doi.org/10.2337/dc11-0471

6  Action to Control Cardiovascular Risk in Diabetes Study Group, Gerstein, H. C., Miller, M. E., Byington, R. P, et.al. (2008). Effects of intensive glucose lowering in type 2 diabetes. *The New England journal of medicine*, *358*(24), 2545–2559. https://doi.org/10.1056/NEJMoa0802743

7  Diabetes Control and Complications Trial Research Group, Nathan, D. M., Genuth, S., Lachin, J., Cleary, P., Crofford, O., Davis, M., Rand, L., & Siebert, C. (1993). The effect of intensive treatment of diabetes on the development and progression of long-term complications in insulin-dependent diabetes mellitus. *The New England journal of medicine*, *329*(14), 977–986. https://doi.org/10.1056/NEJM199309303291401

8  Intensive blood-glucose control with sulphonylureas or insulin compared with conventional treatment and risk of complications in patients with type 2 diabetes (UKPDS 33). UK Prospective Diabetes Study (UKPDS) Group. (1998). *Lancet (London, England)*, *352*(9131), 837–853.

9  Ohkubo Y, Kishikawa H, Araki E, Miyata T, Isami S, et al. Intensive insulin therapy prevents the progression of diabetic microvascular complications in Japanese patients with non-insulin-dependent diabetes mellitus—a randomized prospective 6-year study. Diabetes Res Clin Pract 1995;28:103-17.

10  Holman, R. R., Paul, S. K., Bethel, M. A., Neil, H. A., & Matthews, D. R. (2008). Long-term follow-up after tight control of blood pressure in type 2 diabetes. *The New England journal of medicine*, *359*(15), 1565–1576. https://doi.org/10.1056/NEJMoa0806359

11  Raccah, D., Huet, D., Dib, A., Joseph, F., Landers, B., Escalada, J., & Schmitt, H. (2017). Review of basal-plus insulin regimen options for simpler insulin intensification in people with Type 2 diabetes mellitus. *Diabetic medicine: a journal of the British Diabetic Association*, *34*(9), 1193–1204. https://doi.org/10.1111/dme.13390

12  Ligthelm, R. J., Mouritzen, U., Lynggaard, H., Landin-Olsson, et. al., (2006). Biphasic insulin aspart given thrice daily is as efficacious as a basal-bolus insulin regimen with four daily injections: a randomised open-label parallel group four months comparison in patients with type 2 diabetes. *Experimental and clinical endocrinology & diabetes: official journal, German Society of Endocrinology [and] German Diabetes Association*, *114*(9), 511–519. https://doi.org/10.1055/s-2006-924424

# CHAPTER 6
# Management of Diabetes Complications

*Success is not final; failure is not fatal: It is the courage to continue that counts.*
**Winston Churchill**

Despite the evolution of the diabetes treatment modalities, the complications of diabetes continue to present major clinical and health economic challenges today. The increasing complications with complex multisystem effects, prolonged admissions, and the increased use of limited medical resources remain the major challenges to any healthcare systems in the world.

## Classification of Diabetes Complications

Diabetes complications are essentially classified into two major categories—*acute* and *chronic*.

### Acute Complications

- Infections
- Hypoglycaemia
- Hyperglycaemic states
    - Diabetic ketoacidosis (DKA)
    - Hyperglycaemic Hyperosmolar state (HHS)
    - Transient Hyperglycaemic states (Somogyi effect and dawn phenomena)

### Chronic Complications

Uncontrolled long-standing diabetes affects the vascular system and causes vascular complications. Therefore, the chronic complications are classified as either microvascular or macrovascular complications, depending on the size and calibre of the vessels:

- Microvascular complications
    - Retinopathy
    - Neuropathy
    - Nephropathy

- Macrovascular complications
    - Stroke
    - Myocardial infarction
    - Peripheral vascular disease

**Complications of Diabetes Mellitus**

1. Acute complications
   - Infections
   - Hypoglycaemia
   - Hyperglycaemic states

2. Chronic complications
   - Microvascular
   - Macrovascular

## Management of Acute Complications of Diabetes

### Infections

Diabetic patients are immunosuppressed and are, therefore, prone to all different kinds of infections, with the potential for quick deterioration, prolonged healing, and delayed recovery. Any infections in diabetic patients must be treated aggressively and appropriately according to local antimicrobial guidelines.

If treatment is delayed, infections can lead to further complications of hyperglycaemic states (DKA and HHS), sepsis, and death.

### Hypoglycaemia

Hypoglycaemia is a state of low plasma glucose associated with symptoms. The plasma glucose level of 3.9 mmo/l (70 mg/dl) is taken as the lower level by which symptoms occur. However, diabetics with chronic hyperglycaemia will also present with symptoms at higher levels of plasma glucose, and that level defines their threshold for hypoglycaemia.

Hypoglycaemia can happen in both diabetic and non-diabetic patients. It is more common among diabetic patients treated with insulin, sulphonylureas, and the glitinides than those with other treatments. Furthermore, it is three to four times more common in T1DM compared with T2DM and is more prevalent among those with long duration of diabetes. [1, 2]

The body's warning system can detect hypoglycaemia through clusters of symptoms that alert the person to take remedial measures (eat/drink) to alleviate the hypoglycaemic symptoms.

These symptoms are often grouped as:

- *General symptoms* (nausea, dizziness and collapse, low mood, and lethargy)
- *Sympathetic/autonomic symptoms* (sweating, tremor, palpitation, tachycardia, agitation, nervousness, and hunger)
- *Neuroglycopenic symptoms* (difficulty in concentration, slowed speech, slowed thinking and lack of coordination, aggressive behaviour, focal neurological deficits mimicking stroke, seizures, and loss of consciousness)

## Diagnosis of Hypoglycemia by Whipple's Triad

The diagnosis of hypoglycemia is based on a triad named after Dr Allen O. Whipple.[3] These include symptoms of hypoglycemia with a low blood glucose and relief of symptoms on treatment.

*Whipple's triad involves:*

- Low blood glucose level
- Symptoms of hypoglycemia at the time of the low glucose level
- Symptom relief with treatment of hypoglycemia

## Management of Hypoglycaemia

Management is based on severity as defined by the International Hypoglycaemic Study Group (IHSG). [4]

- Mild hypoglycaemia is characterised by sugar level of
- Moderate hypoglycaemia is characterised by both autonomic and neuroglycopenic symptoms and individuals can self-treat.
- Severe hypoglycaemia is characterised by unconsciousness and requires the assistance of another person to treat either with glucagon injection or glucose infusion or carbohydrate.

## Hypoglycaemic Unawareness

The counter-regulatory responses (warning system) to hypoglycaemia, which is characterised by the release of adrenaline, glucagon, GH, and cortisol, are blunted in some patients with recurrent hypoglycaemia as shown in Figure 6.1. These patients are not aware of the low level of their blood glucose. [5] This group of diabetics has:

- Frequent hypoglycaemic episodes
- Long-standing diabetes
- Tightly controlled diabetes

Patients with hypoglycaemic unawareness will lose their *physical* and *mood* symptoms of hypoglycaemia but do not lose their neuroglycopenic symptoms. Therefore, symptoms such as difficulty in concentration, slowed speech, slowed thinking, and lack of coordination could be used to recognise hypoglycaemia and initiate correction. It requires the patient's understanding of symptoms of neuroglycopenia, insulin effect, and carbohydrate intact. Surely this does not protect the patient during sleep, and appropriate adjustment is required to prevent any hypoglycaemia during sleep. [6]

Failure to treat hypoglycaemic episodes will lead to hypoglycaemic autonomic failure (HAF), commonly known as the hypoglycaemic unawareness. This relates to the adage 'hypoglycaemia begets hypoglycaemia'. The main mechanism for unawareness is not known. [7]

To treat and reverse this stage of HAF requires the 'rule of 3':

- Monitor blood glucose ≥ three times per day.
- Prevent hypoglycaemia for ≥ three days.
- Do this for three weeks.

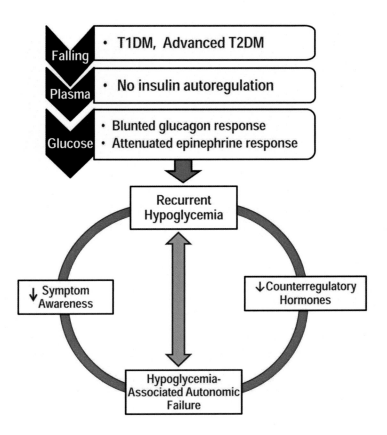

**Figure 6.1** Pathophysiology of hypoglycaemic autonomic failure whereby "Hypoglycaemia begets hypoglycaemia". Reproduced from Samuel Dagogo-Jack; Philip E. Cryer, MD: Seminal Contributions to the Understanding of Hypoglycaemia and Glucose Counter regulation and the Discovery of HAAF (Cryer Syndrome). *Diabetes Care* 1 December 2015; 38 (12): 2193–2199. https://doi.org/10.2337/dc15-0533

---

**Hypoglycaemic unawareness is characterised by a cycle of recurrent hypoglycaemia with maladaptive memory and habituation. It is a hypoglycaemic autonomic failure.**

---

## Hyperglycaemic States

### Diabetes Ketoacidosis (DKA)

DKA can occur in both type 1 and the type 2 diabetes mellitus. According to the 2013 Joint British Society Guideline,[8] DKA consists of a biochemical triad of:

- Ketonemia (Ketosis) ≥3 mmo/l or significant ketonuria ≥2+ on standard urine dipsticks
- Hyperglycaemia (BG >11 or known DM)
- Acidaemia (bicarbonate <15 and or venous pH <7.3)

**DKA is characterised by a triad of:**

1. Hyperglycaemia
2. Ketonemia
3. Acidaemia

## Pathophysiology

DKA is usually triggered by an infection or a stressful body situation such as inflammation, stroke, trauma, and myocardial infarction. Counter-regulatory hormones such as adrenaline, cortisol, glucagon, and growth hormone are released, which increase glycogenolysis from the liver, increases gluconeogenesis from the proteins from the muscles, and increase the fatty acid breakdown from triglycerides. Metabolism is shifted from glucose oxidation to fatty acid metabolism, resulting in the production of ketones (acetone, beta-hydroxybutyric and acetoacetate).

Excessive ketones then cause metabolic ketoacidosis and are filtered through the urine. The beta-hydroxybutyric can cause nausea and vomiting, further aggravating fluid loss and acidosis.

A third of patients can present with clinical features overlapping between the DKA and the HHS state (overlap cases). This means the two states of the uncontrolled diabetes differ in the magnitude of dehydration and severity of acidosis. [9]

## Management of DKA

The Joint British Diabetes Society guideline 2018 advises using fixed-rate insulin infusion (FRII) at 0.1 unit/kg for those with significant acidosis (venous HCO3 <15 mmol/L and/or venous pH <7.3, associated with ketonemia (ketone ≥3mmol/L on ketone meter or ketonuria ++ or more on standard urine dipstick).

Patients with ketonemia but *without* acidosis must not be given IV insulin. Hydration with subcutaneous insulin can be considered.

If blood ketones are not falling by at least 0.5 mmol/L per hour *or* venous bicarbonate isn't rising by at least 3 mmol/L per hour *or* CBG is not falling by at least 3 mmol/L per hour, increase insulin infusion rate by 1.0 unit per hour until the fall meets the target rates.

Change to variable-rate insulin infusion (VRII) when ketonemia is 0.6mmol/L and HCO3 >15, pH >7.3, and patients starts to eat and drink. Continue basal insulin and allow VRII to go for two hours before stopping. [10]

## Fluid Resuscitation in DKA

Most patients come in severely dehydrated due to infection, lack of fluid intake, fever, and humid hot weather in summer in the temperate countries and in the tropical countries. Follow fluid prescription as per the joint British Diabetic Society Guidelines. A quick simple way is to consider patient profile and rehydrate safely with intravenous fluid up to safe hydration status. Regular monitoring of fluid status is advised to prevent complications of fluid overload such as the cerebral oedema, ARDS, and heart failure.

## Electrolyte Management in DKA

Potassium is usually elevated in DKA. Do not give KCL if potassium is above 5.6mmol/l. Rather, observe, monitor, and replace when it falls. If potassium is <5.6mmol/L consider replacement with insulin in saline infusion.

## Education in DKA

Reinforcing patient education on diabetes and its complications is important on every occasion of patients' visits, either in ill health or during normal reviews. Apply 'sick day rules'— specific education, teaching patients to increase their insulin dosages, turn up to the hospital when they feel sick, or monitor their urinary ketones with a dipstick. They must be told to continue to drink water and if diarrhoea and vomiting persist for twenty-four hours, then they must stop their metformin and present to the hospital.

---

### DKA insulin treatment threshold (insulin dose 0.1units/kg/hr)

- Hyperglycaemia: BG >11.1
- Ketosis: Ketonuria ≥2+ or Ketonemia ≥3+
- Acidaemia: Venous HCO3 < 15, or pH < 7.3

### Target success rate

- Hyperglycaemia: BG drop by 5mmol/L/hr
- Ketosis: Ketone drop by 0.5mmol/L/hr
- Acidaemia: HCO3 rise by 3mmol/L/hr

### Insulin escalation dose (1 unit/kg/hr if target not met)

### Weaned off FRII to VRII when:

- Ketones: 0.6mmol/L
- Acidaemia: HCO3 >15, pH >7.3
- Eating and drinking

---

## Hyperosmolar hyperglycaemic state (HHS)

Hyperosmolar hyperglycaemic state (HHS) is a serious acute complication of diabetes with an estimated mortality of 10 to 20% higher than DKA. It was previously known as a hyperosmolar hyperglycaemic nonketotic coma (HONK). But the term has been changed to HHS because only 20% of those experiencing HHS have a real coma. It can happen in both types of diabetes but is more common in T2DM and more frequent among the elderly.

HHS is characterised by: [11-13]

- hyperglycaemia
- hyperosmolarity
- severe dehydration +/- focal or global neurologic deficits
- without significant ketoacidosis

According to the consensus statement published by the American Diabetes Association, the diagnostic features of HHS may include the following: [12-14]

- Plasma glucose level of 600 mg/dL (33.3 mmol/l) or greater
- Effective serum osmolality of 320 mOsm/kg or greater
- Profound dehydration, up to an average of 9L
- Serum pH greater than 7.30
- Bicarbonate concentration greater than 15 mmol/L
- Small ketonuria and absent-to-low ketonemia
- Some alteration in consciousness

## Pathophysiology

The underlying mechanism of HHS is a relative or absolute reduction in effective circulating insulin with a concomitant elevation of counter-regulatory hormones (epinephrine, cortisol, growth hormone, and glucagon).

Decreased renal clearance and decreased peripheral utilisation of glucose lead to hyperglycaemia. Hyperglycaemia and hyperosmolarity result in an osmotic diuresis and an osmotic shift of fluid to the intravascular space, resulting in further intracellular dehydration. This diuresis also leads to loss of electrolytes, such as sodium and potassium.

Unlike patients with DKA, patients with HHS do not develop significant ketoacidosis, but the reason for this is not known. Contributing factors likely include the availability of insulin in amounts sufficient to inhibit ketogenesis but insufficient to prevent hyperglycaemia. Additionally, hyperosmolarity itself may decrease lipolysis, limiting the amount of free fatty acids available for ketogenesis. In addition, the levels of the counter-regulatory hormones are found to be lower in patients with HHS than in those with DKA.

## Management in HHS

### Fluid resuscitation

Normal saline infusion using basic fluid resuscitation protocol as per the British Diabetes Society Guideline is advised with the objective of 'safe rehydration to normal hydration status' based on the patient clinical profile.

Monitor fluid levels—not to overload and not to underload. Beware of acute deterioration in patients recovering well and suddenly deteriorating with confusion and/or agitation. This could be cerebral oedema.

### Insulin treatment

Patients who have been on either intermediate and or basal insulin treatment before presentation must maintain their subcutaneous insulin treatment. Insulin treatment must only be commenced in newly diagnosed HHS if significant ketonuria (++) or ketonemia (3+) is present.

- Treat/address the precipitating factor—antibiotics if infection but blood culture and other appropriate investigations need to be done beforehand.
- Thromboembolic prophylaxis with enoxaparin or low molecular weight heparin be initiated.

- The pathophysiology of DKA and HHS are similar: Both have absolute and or relative reduction in effective circulating insulin with a concomitant elevation of counter-regulatory hormones (epinephrine, cortisol, growth hormone, and glucagon) triggered by infection, inflammation, and/or trauma.
- DKA patients resort to fatty acid metabolism to produce ketones as an alternate fuel to glucose, whilst hyperglycaemia in HHS leads to osmotic diuresis with dehydration and serum hyperosmolarity.
- The reason for HHS not developing ketones is not known but is assumed to be due to availability of insulin in amounts sufficient to inhibit ketogenesis but insufficient to prevent hyperglycaemia.

**Transient Hyperglycaemic States**

Healthcare workers often confuse between the two transient states of morning hyperglycaemia; Somogyi hyperglycaemia a bona fide marker of raised counter regulatory hormones in the morning and Dawn hyperglycaemia, a marker of nocturnal weaning effect of insulin.

### Somogyi Effect

The Somogyi effect is a state of morning hyperglycaemia that resists insulin therapy and requires additional insulin doses. It is named after a Hungarian-born professor, Michael Somogyi.

It is controversial, as it is deemed to be a reactive hyperglycaemia secondary to an episode of nocturnal hypoglycaemia among patients treated with insulin.

The Somogyi effect is now thought to be due to an increase in morning cortisol level, and other counter-regulatory hormones and is not a marker of nocturnal hypoglycaemia but, rather, a marker of nocturnal hyperglycaemia. [15]

### Dawn Phenomenon

Morning hyperglycaemia secondary to weaning of nocturnal insulin effect is known as the Dawn Phenomenon. Appropriate insulin type can be prescribed in optimal doses to control this phenomenon.

## Management of Chronic Complications of Diabetes

The strategies involved in the management of the chronic complications of diabetes are to prevent the deterioration and improve the quality of life among the diabetic population. These strategies form the basis of tertiary prevention.

## The Pathophysiology of Chronic Complications

The exact cause of the pathophysiology of the chronic complications of diabetes are not entirely known. However, several potential pathological mechanisms have been proposed, as shown in **Figure 6.2**. Although a deep exploration of these mechanisms are beyond the intent of this book, several of them, in brief, are:

- Polyol pathway—non-enzymatic glycosylation of proteins and lipids
- Protein kinase C (PKC) activation
- Increased flux through the hexosamine pathway
- Increased oxidative stress

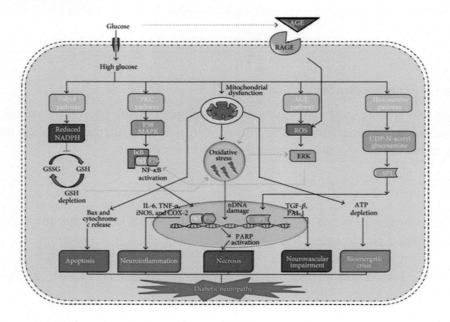

**Figure 6.2** Different pathological pathways leading to chronic diabetic complications. Reproduced from Sandireddy, R., Yerra, V. G., Areti, A., Komirishetty, P., & Kumar, A. (2014). Neuroinflammation and oxidative stress in diabetic neuropathy: futuristic strategies based on these targets. *International journal of endocrinology, 2014*, 674987. https://doi.org/10.1155/2014/674987

Polyol Pathway

One of these important mechanisms is the polyol pathway shown in **Figure 6.3**. Tissues in the body are either responsive or non-responsive to insulin. Insulin-dependent tissues include liver and the muscles, whilst the brain, eyes, kidneys, and the nerves are insulin independent.

Excess glucose unused for energy production enters the polyol pathway—a pathway that leads to the reduced production of the reducing agents NADPH and NAD and increased sorbitol production. This process of glucose catalysation to sorbitol is done by an enzyme called aldolase reductase. Therefore aldose reductase inhibitors are used to improve nerve conduction.

The reduction in the reducing agents results in the reduced synthesis of glutathione, nitric oxide, and myoinositol, which are required for the normal function of the nerves.

Sorbitol, on the other hand, does not cross the cell membrane and, so, accumulates and draws water, causing osmotic stress on the insulin-independent tissues. Further, sorbitol forms glycation with the proteins and the collagen on the vascular walls, affecting the normal physiology of the endothelial cells.

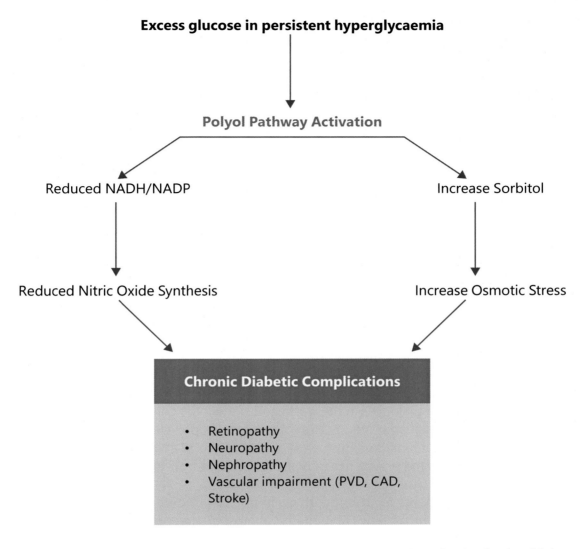

**Figure 6.3** The Polyol Pathway. Activation leads to increased sorbitol production by the aldolase enzyme. Sorbitol induces osmotic lysis by disrupting cell wall membrane of insulin-independent tissue cells and increases osmotic stress leading to chronic complications of diabetes.

Redox imbalance stress in diabetes mellitus: Role of the polyol pathway

### Advanced glycation end products (AGEs)

Excess glucose reacts with proteins, nucleotides, and lipids; and these results in advanced glycation end products (AGEs). They may have a role in disrupting the integrity of neurons and repair mechanisms by interfering with neuronal cell metabolism and axonal transport.

### Oxidative stress

There is increased production of free radicals in diabetes. The mechanism of damage is not fully understood. They may cause direct damage to blood vessels, leading to nerve ischemia and facilitating AGE reactions.

**Several pathological pathways lead to end products causing chronic diabetes complications:**

- **Polyol pathway**. Decreased reducing agents reduces vascular molecules, which maintain vascular wall health. Increased sorbitol facilitates vascular wall degeneration.
- **Advanced glycation end products (AGEPs)**. Non enzymatic glycation of lipids and proteins called Schiff base with excess glucose in a process called Browning leads to transient glycated products. Rearrangements lead to early advanced glycated products called Amadori type advanced early GEP. With complex reactions, these finally become AGEP, which are irreversible and destroy the vascular walls.
- **PKC pathway**. Increased intracellular glucose increases diacylglycerol (DAC), which activates PKC. PKC reduces vascular nitric oxide and upregulation of proinflammatory genes and vascular adhesion molecules.
- **Hexosamine pathway**. Shunting of excess glucose into this pathway leads to phosphorylation of serine/threonine—an important step in upregulation of many endothelial enzymes—leading to reduced endothelial vascular nitric oxide and increased transforming growth factor-1.

## Management of Microvascular Complications

### Retinopathy

Diabetes is a leading cause of blindness in the world and is the most common cause of visual loss in the United Kingdom and is rising in Papua New Guinea. Although, the prevalence of diabetes retinopathy has declined with insulin therapy, it remains extremely high—between 32 and 59%. Given the expected rise in diabetes in the next decades, the prevalence of diabetic retinopathy is expected to rise proportionately.

Screening of all diabetic patients for retinopathy is important to detect, prevent, and treat all sight-threatening maculopathy and proliferative retinopathy, as most unscreened patients remain asymptomatic until they present with proliferative retinopathy or macular oedema.

Therefore, it is imperative to control blood sugar, hypertension, and dyslipidaemia among diabetic patients and monitor, diagnose, and treat their retinopathy in the early stages to prevent blindness.

### Pathophysiology of Diabetic Retinopathy

Chronic hyperglycaemia impairs the autoregulation of retinal blood flow by increasing the retinal flow. This increases the shear stress on the retinal blood vessels, which may be a stimulus for micro dilatations, vascular leakages, the production of vasoactive substances, and increased fluid accumulation in the outer layers of the retina, resulting in macular oedema.

### Stages of Retinopathy and Treatment Approaches[16]

Non-proliferative diabetic retinopathy—non sight threatening

- *No apparent diabetic retinopathy (DR)*
  No evidence of early stages of diabetes retinopathy
    – Full fundoscopy yearly and no referral to ophthalmologist
    – Aggressive glycaemic, blood pressure, and lipid control

- *Mild non-proliferative diabetes retinopathy*
  Evidence of microaneurysm
    – Full fundoscopy in six to twelve months and no referral to ophthalmologist
    – Continue control of blood sugar, blood pressure, and lipids

- *Moderate non-proliferative diabetes retinopathy*
  Evidence of microaneurysm plus other signs (dots and blots, hard exudates, and cotton wool spots) but less than severe non-proliferative DR
    – Full fundoscopy in three to six months but no referral to ophthalmologist
    – Continue optimal management of risk factors.

- *Severe non-proliferative diabetes retinopathy*
  Anyone of these signs—intraretinal haemorrhages (≥20 in each quadrant), venous beading in two quadrants or intraretinal microvascular in one quadrant with no proliferation
    – Full fundoscopy in three months and referral to ophthalmologist
    – Continue optimal management of risk factors

Sight-threatening Retinopathy.

- *Proliferative diabetic retinopathy*
  Severe non-proliferative DR or either one of neovascularisation or vitreous/preretinal haemorrhages
    – Referral to ophthalmologist for photocoagulation

- *Maculopathy—macular oedema*
  Circinate formation of hard exudates around the macular area
  Macular oedema is not detected by direct ophthalmoscopy.
    – Referral to ophthalmologist for photocoagulation in focal maculopathy and/or intravitreal injections of ranibizumab or bevacizumab in diffuse maculopathy may be more effective at stabilising or improving vision on their own or in combination with laser photocoagulation.

### Stages of Diabetic Retinopathy

1. Non-proliferative diabetic retinopathy (NPDR)
   - Mild
   - Moderate
   - Severe
2. Proliferative diabetic retinopathy (PDR)
3. Diabetic maculopathy (DM)

## Photocoagulation

Photocoagulation is the treatment of choice for the diabetic proliferative and maculopathies. There are two types of photocoagulations—*focal* or *diffuse* (*panretinal* or *scattering*). Based on the stages of retinopathies and the degree of risks the specific type of diffuse photocoagulation could cause further loss of visual acuity.

There are two forms of photocoagulators, which essentially differ in the wavelength absorption by the haemoglobin: [17]

- Krypton red photocoagulator is useful in treatment when the neovascularisation is closer than 200 µm but not under the fovea because of its ability to spare the inner retina by its virtual lack of absorption by haemoglobin.
- Argon laser photocoagulator is the conventional one with blue-green wavelength. The green wavelength is absorbed by haemoglobin and, thus, may damage the retina, whilst the blue wavelength is absorbed by the macular xanthophyll and results in foveal damage.

### Anti-Vascular Endothelial Growth Factor (anti-VEGF) Injection Maculopathy

Diffuse diabetic maculopathy may respond relatively poorly to laser treatment. The Royal Collage of Ophthalmology (UK) recommends intravitreal injections of ranibizumab or bevacizumab. These could be more effective at stabilising or improving vision on their own or in combination with laser photocoagulation. Research to determine the optimum frequency and duration of injections is ongoing.

### Vitreoretinal Surgery

Vitreoretinal surgery may be required for a minority of patients who develop severe diabetic eye disease.

### Neuropathy

There are several types of diabetic neuropathies, all caused by prolonged uncontrolled blood sugar levels:

- Peripheral neuropathy
- Mononeuritis
- Autonomic neuropathy

### Peripheral Neuropathy

Patients present classically with 'stocking glove' distribution of sensory loss in the feet and hands respectively. The earliest signs could be either positive (tingling or pain) or negative (numbness or paraesthesia). Screening with monofilament at pressure points can detect these early stages of peripheral neuropathy, and appropriate management can be instituted in combination with aggressive glycaemic, blood pressure, and lipid control.

The complications of peripheral neuropathy such as the neuropathic pain can be managed with neuropathic pain medications such as amitriptyline, pregabalin or gabapentin. The neuropathic ulcers are often difficult to manage and therefore would require podiatric support.

### Mononeuritis

Mononeuritis, also known as mononeuropathy, is a form of peripheral neuropathy where only one nerve is affected. If several nerves are affected, then it's called mononeuritis multiplex or multifocal neuropathies. Both peripheral nerves and cranial nerves can be affected and often in different regions. Management is difficult and occasionally involves the use of steroids and immunosuppressants.

### Autonomic Neuropathy

This subtype of diabetic neuropathy is quite extensive, and management is based on the organ function affected. Among the organs affected and possible treatments:

- Gastroparesis can present with early satiety, postprandial bloating, nausea, and vomiting. It can be treated with prokinetics such as metoclopramide and or cisapride.

- Enteric neuropathy affects intestinal motility and leads to various symptoms, such as nocturnal diarrhoea, constipation, intestinal pain, and abdominal distension and can even simulate bowel obstruction. Management can be difficult and is symptomatic.
- Upper and lower motor neuron lesions of bladder can lead to urinary retention (overflow incontinence) or dribbling incontinence. These can be managed accordingly with alpha 1 receptor antagonists (prazosin, doxazocin) and anticholinergics (oxybutynin, solifenacin, and mirabegron) respectively.
- Erectile dysfunction is one of the earliest precursors of autonomic neuropathies. Management can be aided by erection pills.
- Loss of BP autoregulation results in drop in postural BP. It can be managed with fludrocortisone and or midodrine hydrochloride.

## Nephropathy[18, 19]

Diabetic nephropathy is a clinical syndrome characterised by the following:

- Persistent albuminuria (>300 mg/d or >200 μg/min) that is confirmed on at least two occasions three to six months apart
- Progressive decline in the glomerular filtration rate (GFR)
- Elevated arterial blood pressure

### Pathophysiology

Three major histologic changes occur in the glomeruli of persons with diabetic nephropathy. First, mesangial expansion is directly induced by hyperglycaemia, perhaps via increased matrix production or glycosylation of matrix proteins. Second, thickening of the glomerular basement membrane (GBM) occurs. Third, glomerular sclerosis is caused by intraglomerular hypertension (induced by dilatation of the afferent renal artery or from ischemic injury induced by hyaline narrowing of the vessels supplying the glomeruli). These different histologic patterns appear to have similar prognostic significance. The basement membrane becomes thicker, which is quite different from other causes of chronic renal diseases.

### Rationale for Screening for Diabetes Nephropathy

Diabetes nephropathy is a common complication of diabetes that, with current treatment is easily preventable with screening and appropriate early treatment. It's important because of its effects on the lives of patients in terms of their morbidity and mortality and, importantly, the costs involved in managing chronic renal failure (CRF), leading to end-stage renal failure (ESRF). Personal costs and the costs to the healthcare systems have greatly increased over the years, and this requires prevention (both primary and secondary).

For T1DM, screening is generally recommended at five years after diagnosis. But since many patients—as high as 18%—can have proteinuria before five years and puberty as an independent factor for proteinuria, screening for T1DM must start one year after diagnosis.

Screening for T2DM must be initiated at the time of diagnosis. Annual screening is instituted for both types of diabetes without micro-albuminuria.

### Methods of Screening

There are many techniques available for screening diabetic nephropathy, but standard, cost-effective, and readily available screening tests include testing patients' urine for evidence of proteinuria. The arduous twenty-four-hour urine is cumbersome and is rarely done. However, three screening tests are commonly used for detecting urinary proteinuria—the basic urinary dipstick, PCR, and ACR.

a. *Urinary dipsticks*
- A crude, less sensitive screening test
- More readily available at bedside, in the clinics and the wards than the other two below

b. *Protein–creatinine ratio*
- Urinary protein/creatinine >45mg/mmol
- Can be used as screening method but has lower sensitivity than ACR
- Used as a monitoring tool of diabetic nephropathy

c. *Albumin-creatinine ratio*
- Albumin-creatinine >30mg/mmol
- Is more sensitive than PCR
- Used in screening, diagnosis, and monitoring of diabetic nephropathy

An eGFR calculator online should be used to assess the renal function for staging purpose. Start patients early on ACE-I or ARB if ACE-I is contraindicated for all diabetic patients for renoprotection.

> **Screening Tools for Early Diabetic Nephropathy**
>
> 1. Urine dipsticks
> 2. Protein-creatinine ratio
> 3. Albumin-creatinine ratio

## Stages of Diabetic Nephropathy

Alterations in renal structure and function occur at the outset of diabetes. It is a chronic process that continues unabated though at slower rates with treatment.

With accumulating evidence over the last several decades, diabetic renal changes have been classified. [19] These provide important clinical, prognostic, and management information.

### Stage 1

- Early hyperfunction and hypertrophy
- Increased urinary albumin excretion
- Changes are at least partly reversible by insulin treatment
- Renal function tests are normal, GFR normal >90 ml/1.74 m$^2$

### Stage 2

- Develops silently over many years and is characterised by morphologic lesions without signs of clinical disease
- The function is characterized by increased GFR, and biopsy shows renal lesions
- Renal function tests normal, GFR 60–90 ml/1.74 m$^3$

### Stage 3

- Incipient diabetic nephropathy is the forerunner of overt diabetic nephropathy

- Its main manifestation is abnormally elevated urinary albumin excretion, as measured by radioimmunoassay
- Renal function tests abnormal

*Stage 3A*

- GFR 45–60 ml/1.74 m$^2$
- Renal anaemia sets in (erythropoietin deficiency), erythropoietin must be started in this stage

*Stage 3B*

- GFR 30–45ml/1.74 m$^2$

*Stage 4*

- Overt diabetic nephropathy
- The classic entity characterised by persistent proteinuria (>0.5 g/ 24 h). When the associated high blood pressure is left untreated, renal function (GFR) declines, the mean fall rate being around 1 ml/min/mo. Long-term antihypertensive treatment reduces the fall rate by about 60% and, thus, postpones uraemia considerably.
- GFR 15–30 ml/1.74 m$^2$
- Renal replacement therapy must be started in this phase

*Stage 5—end-stage renal failure*

- End-stage renal failure with uraemia due to diabetic nephropathy. As many as 25% of the population presently entering end-stage renal failure programs in the United States are diabetic.
- Dialysis as bridge to transplant
- Renal transplant as definitive treatment

### Stages of Diabetic Nephropathy

1. Stage I—eGFR >90 mls/1.74 m$^3$
2. Stage II—eGFR 60–90 mls/1.74 m$^3$
3. Stage III
   - IIIA—eGFR 45–60 ml/1.74 m$^2$
   - IIIB—eGFR 30–45 ml/1.74 m$^2$
4. Stage IV—eGFR 15–30 ml/1.74 m$^2$
5. Stage V—eGFR < 15 ml/1.74 m$^3$

## Management of Macrovascular Complications

### Stroke

Diabetes has a detrimental effect on the arterial blood vessels, including cerebral vessels. It contributes to strokes independently and in association with other risk factors. It increases the relative risks of ischemic strokes. [20] Ischemic strokes presenting within three and a half hours at any stroke serviced hospitals can be thrombolysed with alteplase according to local protocols.

## Coronary Artery Diseases (CAD)

Diabetes can affect the coronary vessels as well as the myocardium, causing both acute coronary syndromes and diabetic cardiomyopathy. Diabetic associated coronary artery disease (CAD) has a different phenotype compared to non-diabetic CAD. The lesions are diffuse, long, tortuous, and friable and are often difficult to stent. They require highly potent antiplatelet Prasugrel pre- and post-stenting with second- and third-generation drug eluting stents. Most with dual vessel diseases are way more likely to undergo CABG than stenting. Although CABG has increased two-year mortality, it has been shown to reduce mortality significantly five years post-surgery compared with PCI patients. [21]

Diabetic patients presenting with AMI must be given insulin infusion over twenty-four hours, followed by subcutaneous injections for three months. This has been shown to reduce mortality.[22] However, extending beyond three months has not shown any benefits.[23]

## Peripheral Vascular Disease (PVD)

PVD is characterised clinically by the loss of toe hairs, cold feet, reduced dorsalis pedis and anterior tibial pulses, and callous formation on toes. Vascular claudication is the graphic presentation. However, most patients may be diagnosed with simple bedside test called the ankle-brachial index (ABI), which is the ratio of systolic ankle blood pressure divided by brachial systolic blood pressure. The ratio is read as shown by **Table 6.1**.

| ABI Value | Interpretation | Recommendation |
|---|---|---|
| Greater than 1.4 | Calcification/Vessel Hardening | Refer to Vascular Specialist |
| **1.0 – 1.4** | **Normal** | **None** |
| **0.9 – 1.0** | **Borderline** | **None** |
| **0.8 – 0.9** | **Some Arterial Disease** | **Treat Risk Factors** |
| 0.5 – 0.8 | Moderate Arterial Disease | Refer to Vascular Specialist |
| Less than 0.5 | Severe Arterial Disease | Refer to Vascular Specialist |

**Table 6.1** Interpretation of the ankle-brachial Index

## Key Messages:

- **Management of acute complications are in the realm of acute and emergency medicine.**
- **Management of the chronic complications involves multidisciplinary teams input.**
- **Optimising care in this subgroup of diabetic patients is very important to facilitate and promote independence and improve quality of life.**

# References:

1   UK Hypoglycaemia Study Group (2007). Risk of hypoglycaemia in types 1 and 2 diabetes: effects of treatment modalities and their duration. *Diabetologia, 50*(6), 1140–1147. https://doi.org/10.1007/s00125-007-0599-y

2   Donnelly, L. A., Morris, A. D., Frier, B. M., Ellis, J. D., Donnan, P. T., Durrant, R., Band, M. M., Reekie, G., Leese, G. P., & DARTS/MEMO Collaboration (2005). Frequency and predictors of hypoglycaemia in Type 1 and insulin-treated Type 2 diabetes: a population-based study. *Diabetic medicine: a journal of the British Diabetic Association, 22*(6), 749–755. https://doi.org/10.1111/j.1464-5491.2005.01501.x

3   Fischel AH. Hypoglycemia diagnosis. A three - step approach. Whipple's Triad. http://www.endocrineweb.com/conditions/hypoglycemia/hypoglycemia-diagnosis

4   International Hypoglycemia Study Group (IHSG) Classification of Hypoglycemia https://ihsgonline.com/understanding-hypoglycaemia/definition)

5   American Diabetes Association. Hypoglycemia. http://www.diabetes.org/living-with-diabetes/treatment-and-care/blood-glucose-control/hypoglycemia-low-blood.html

6   Joslin Diabetes Center. Stay Healthy with Diabetes. http://www.joslin.org/info/what_can_i_do_to_prevent_serious_hypoglycemic_episodes_when_I_am_hypoglycemic_unaware.html

7   de Galan, B. E., Schouwenberg, B. J., Tack, C. J., & Smits, P. (2006). Pathophysiology and management of recurrent hypoglycaemia and hypoglycaemia unawareness in diabetes. *The Netherlands journal of medicine, 64*(8), 269–279.

8   Diabetes UK. Joint British Diabetes Societies Inpatient Care Group: The Management of diabetic ketoacidosis in adults https://www.diabetes.org.uk/Documents/About%20Us/What%20we%20say/Management-of-DKA-241013.pdf

9   Medscape. Diabetic Ketoacidosis. http://emedicine.medscape.com/article/118361-overview

10  The Joint British Diabetes Society Guidelines (2018).2018_addition_DKA_IPC_Pathway.pdf (abcd.care)

11  Nugent B. W. (2005). Hyperosmolar hyperglycemic state. *Emergency medicine clinics of North America, 23*(3), 629–vii. https://doi.org/10.1016/j.emc.2005.03.006

12  Kitabchi, A. E., Umpierrez, G. E., Murphy, M. B.,et.,al. (2001). Management of hyperglycemic crises in patients with diabetes. *Diabetes care, 24*(1), 131–153. https://doi.org/10.2337/diacare.24.1.131

13  Trence, D. L., & Hirsch, I. B. (2001). Hyperglycemic crises in diabetes mellitus type 2. *Endocrinology and metabolism clinics of North America, 30*(4), 817–831. https://doi.org/10.1016/s0889-8529(05)70217-6.

14  Kitabchi, A. E., Umpierrez, G. E., Murphy, M. B., & Kreisberg, R. A. (2006). Hyperglycemic crises in adult patients with diabetes: a consensus statement from the American Diabetes Association. *Diabetes care, 29*(12), 2739–2748. https://doi.org/10.2337/dc06-9916

15  Diabetes UK. Somogy Phenomenon. http://www.diabetes.co.uk/blood-glucose/somogyi-phenomenon.html

16  Royal Collage of Ophthalmologists. Preferred Practice Guideline. Diabetic Retinopathy Screening and Opthalmological Set up in England (2010). *http//*www.rcophth.ac.uk/core/core_picker/download.asp?id=551

17  Baliga RR. 250 Cases in Internal Medicine. 3rd Ed. (2006).Elservier Limited, London

18  Medscape. Diabetes Nephropathy. https://emedicine.medscape.com › article › 238946

19  Mogensen, C. E., Christensen, C. K., & Vittinghus, E. (1983). The stages in diabetic renal disease. With emphasis on the stage of incipient diabetic nephropathy. *Diabetes, 32 Suppl 2*, 64–78. https://doi.org/10.2337/diab.32.2.s64

20  Norrving B, Oxford Textbook of Stroke and Cerebrovascular Disease pp12, Oxford University Press 2013

21  Tam, D. Y., Dharma, C., Rocha, R., Farkouh, M. E.,et.,al.(2020). Long-Term Survival After Surgical or Percutaneous Revascularization in Patients With Diabetes and Multivessel Coronary Disease. *Journal of the American College of Cardiology, 76*(10), 1153–1164. https://doi.org/10.1016/j.jacc.2020.06.052

22  Malmberg K. (1997). Prospective randomised study of intensive insulin treatment on long term survival after acute myocardial infarction in patients with diabetes mellitus. DIGAMI (Diabetes Mellitus, Insulin Glucose Infusion in Acute Myocardial Infarction) Study Group. *BMJ (Clinical research ed.), 314*(7093), 1512–1515. https://doi.org/10.1136/bmj.314.7093.1512

23  Malmberg, K., Norhammar, A., Wedel, H., & Rydén, L. (1999). Glycometabolic state at admission: important risk marker of mortality in conventionally treated patients with diabetes mellitus and acute myocardial infarction: long-term results from the Diabetes and Insulin-Glucose Infusion in Acute Myocardial Infarction (DIGAMI) study. *Circulation, 99*(20), 2626–2632. https://doi.org/10.1161/01.cir.99.20.2626

CHAPTER 7

# Management of Comorbidities in Diabetes

When you hear about those who are seriously affected by the disease, ask a few follow-up questions about their comorbidities, you will hear a constant theme that there are other things going on.
**Larry Lewis**

## Management of Other Cardiovascular Risk Factors in Diabetes Patients

Diabetes has been recognised as a myocardial infarction (MI) equivalent risk about twenty-four years ago. [1] The National Heart, Lung, and Blood Institute (NHLBI), through the National Cholesterol Evaluation Program (NCEP) III guideline, has recognised diabetes as an established CV risk in its 2001 update and recommended diabetes a cardiovascular heart disease equivalent, having similar risk as those with previous MI without diabetes. [2]

Although effective diabetes management is difficult for clinicians, managing comorbidities in diabetes are even more difficult and exhausting. In fact, poor management of comorbidities in diabetes leads to poor diabetes management, and that can further increase the risks of diabetes complications in the long term.

It was in the 1990s that the realisation of management of the comorbidities among the diabetes has led to better outcomes. Therefore, the effective management of the comorbidities, by setting and meeting targets can significantly reduce diabetes complications such as CVD and diabetes nephropathy. This chapter discusses the management of the following comorbidities:

- Blood pressure
- Dyslipidaemia
- Smoking

### Lipid Management

Dyslipidaemia is an established risk factor for acute coronary syndrome. For diabetic patients with normal levels of low-density cholesterol (LDL-C), the risk of CVD increases by three to fivefold compared with the non-diabetic patients. The mechanism for this heightened risk is generally not known but other risk factors, such as the metabolic syndrome and the high number of LDL-C could contribute to this heightened risk.

In 2004, the National Cholesterol Evaluation Program (NCEP) white paper was endorsed by the National Heart, Lung, and Blood Institute (NHLBI), American College of Cardiologists (ACC) and the American Heart Association (AHA). They recommended that, in all diabetic patients, an LDL-C goal of less than 70 mg/dL is a reasonable therapeutic option. [3] The suggestion was based on available clinical trial data such as the Collaborative Atorvastatin Diabetes Study (CARDS trial).

The CARDS trial was a primary preventative study of 2,838 patients with type 2 diabetes who were randomised to atorvastatin 10 mg or placebo. This study was terminated early due to a 37% reduction in major cardiovascular events. [4]

A lower lipid profile was thus recommended, 'the lower the better approach'. Therefore, according to the old Adult Treatment Panel (ATP) III recommendations, patients with diabetes, the lipid targets should be:

- Total cholesterol = < 2.6 mmol/l
- LDL-C = < 1.8 mmol/l
- Non-HDL-C = >1.6 mmol/l
- Triglycerides ≤ 1.7 mmol/l
- Total cholesterol / HDL ratio = under 5.0

The 2014 lipid guideline by ACC/AHA has done away with target setting because of lack of randomised controlled trials and recommends reduction of cholesterol by 50% from its baseline. The EASD/ESC guidelines still maintain lipid targets in management of diabetic patients. One should understand the differences between the AHA/ACC and the ESC/EASD 2014 guidelines on lipid management. Generally, the lower the better approach is the acceptable strategy in lipid management.

Options of management should be in the order of optimal dose of maximum high-intensity statin to reach target. If target is not reached, then add a non-statin like Vytorin to reach the target. The proprotein convertase subtilisin/kexin type 9 (PCSK9) inhibitors, a potent class of anti cholesterol drug is also available and can be used in those who have statin side effects or intolerance and those whose targets are not achieved with statin plus Vytorin combinations.

Fibrates and niacin do have lowering effects of cholesterol and significant improvements in HDL-C but have not been shown to have any clinical benefits.

## Hypertension Management

Hypertension is also an independent risk factor for CVD. It increases the risks of end organ damage if associated with diabetes. Therefore, hypertensive diabetic patients must be treated appropriately and optimally. It has been shown that hypertension treatment reduces cardiovascular outcomes.

The NICE guideline recommends: [5]

- Target BP < 130/80 mmHg for people with end organ damage (kidney, eye, or cardiovascular damage).
- BP target < 140/80 mmHg for those without end organ damage. ADA has also recommended the same target.

These BP targets are different from that of the general population. NICE and the AHA state BP targets for HTN as below:

- People aged under 80 years—lower than 140/90 mmHg
- People aged over 80 years—lower than 150/90 mmHg

### Pharmacotherapy

Diabetic patients with or without hypertension, must be started on ACE-I unless contraindicated. If contraindicated, an ARB-I for hypertension and renoprotective effects can be substitute. [6] Other antihypertensive drugs can be added based on the clinical presentations of the patient using the British Hypertensive Society (BHS) recommendations of A/B or C/D algorithm:

- **A**ngiotensin converting enzyme inhibitors or angiotensin receptor blocker
- **B**eta blocker as mono or dual therapy or
- **C**alcium channel blockers (dihydropyridines, amlodipine or nifedipine)
- **D**iuretics (hydrochlorothiazide or indapamide)

The non-dihydropyridine calcium channel blocker can be considered if blood pressure not reaching target. The SGLT2 receptor antagonists have diuretic effect has also been shown to reduce BP.

## Smoking

Smoking increases cardiovascular diseases by three to fivefold independent of diabetes. It is imperative to advise diabetic patients with this additive risk and help them to cease smoking. The NICE guideline on stopping smoking among people aged twelve years and older is relevant. [7] The advice is discussed in the sections that follow.

### Behavioural support

This can be provided in group or individual settings in the hospital and continued in the communities by community support teams. Mobile phone text messages can be part of the programme.

### Pharmacotherapy

The posology can be referred to the British National Formulary (BNF). Nicotine replacement therapy (NRT) includes both the long- and short-acting therapies. The BNF listed treatments include transdermal patches, gum, inhalation cartridges, sublingual tablets, and a nasal spray.

### e-Cigarettes

It has been shown that patients cease smoking after weaning through e-cigarettes. Evidence is still evolving on this aspect of smoking. Although the risk is lower than traditional smoking, smoking e-cigarettes still has risks. Patients must be advised on this.

## Mnemonic For Optimal Management of Diabetes, Its Complications And The Comorbidities

Managing diabetes, its complications, and the comorbidities correctly, especially by many healthcare workers is quite arduous. This is because of the systemic and the progressive nature of the diabetes complications. Having a pattern or, even better, a mnemonic to remember the management requirements over the long term would allow practitioners to manage diabetic patients appropriately and according to the guidelines.

In the author's experience, a simple mnemonic—**ABCDEFG**—can be very helpful. The mnemonic can be used before discharge after hospitalisation or on reviews so that no management aspects is missed:

**A**

- Hb**A**1c target setting
- **A**nkle-brachial Index
- **A**CE-I (start at the time of diagnosis for renoprotection and/or hypertension) or **A**RB if contraindicated
- **A**spirin

**B**

- **B**lood pressure target < 140/90mmHg
- Blood sugar monitor to optimize treatment

**C**

- **C**holesterol target 1.8 mmol/L (lower is better) (start high intensity statin)
- **C**essation of **c**igarettes and alcohol
- **C**alcium and phosphate level management in diabetic nephropathy

**D**

- Dietary prescription
- Structured **d**ietary education (DAFNE for T1DM, DESMOND for T2DM, and X-PERT for both)

**E**

- **E**ye check—full fundoscopy for evidence of retinopathy
- Baseline **E**CG on diagnosis
- Exercise prescription

**F**

- Foot care—refer to podiatrist and/or tissue viability nurses for care of diabetic foot

**G**

- Guardian medicines (diabetes medicines)

| Optimal Triad of Diabetes Management includes |
| --- |
| 1. Optimal glycaemic control<br>2. Optimal management of complication<br>3. Optimal management of comorbidities |

## Key Messages:

- **Optimal diabetes management include the triad of optimal glycaemic control, optimal management of cardiovascular risk factors to targets in diabetes and the optimal management of the chronic complications.**
- **Remembering the mnemonic 'ABCDEFG' can help in management of diabetes, its chronic complications and the comorbidities.**

## References:

1    Haffner, S. M., Lehto, S., Rönnemaa, T., Pyörälä, K., & Laakso, M. (1998). Mortality from coronary heart disease in subjects with type 2 diabetes and in nondiabetic subjects with and without prior myocardial infarction. *The New England journal of medicine, 339*(4), 229–234. https://doi.org/10.1056/NEJM199807233390404

2    Expert Panel on Detection, Evaluation, and Treatment of High Blood Cholesterol in Adults (2001). Executive Summary of The Third Report of The National Cholesterol Education Program (NCEP) [3]Expert Panel on Detection, Evaluation, And Treatment of High Blood Cholesterol In Adults (Adult Treatment Panel III). *JAMA, 285*(19), 2486–2497. https://doi.org/10.1001/jama.285.19.2486

3    Grundy, S. M., Cleeman, J. I., Merz, C. N.,et. al., & National Heart, Lung, and Blood Institute, American College of Cardiology Foundation, & American Heart Association (2004). Implications of recent clinical trials for the National Cholesterol Education Program Adult Treatment Panel III guidelines. *Circulation, 110*(2), 227–239. https://doi.org/10.1161/01.CIR.0000133317.49796.0E

4    Colhoun, H. M., Thomason, M. J., Mackness, M. I.,et.al., & Collaborative AtoRvastatin Diabetes Study (CARDS) (2002). Design of the Collaborative AtoRvastatin Diabetes Study (CARDS) in patients with type 2 diabetes. *Diabetic medicine: a journal of the British Diabetic Association, 19*(3), 201–211. https://doi.org/10.1046/j.1464-5491.2002.00643.x

5    NICE. Type 2 Diabetes. NICE Guideline. https:// www.nice.org.uk/guidance/cg87. https://www.care.diabetesjournals.org/content/suppl/2014/12/23/38.

6    T. Berl, L. G. Hunsicker, J. B. Lewis, et al., 'Impact of Achieved Blood Pressure on Cardiovascular Outcomes in the Irbesartan Diabetic Nephropathy Trial', *Journal of the American Society of Nephrology*, 16/7 (2005), 2,170–2,179.

7    NICE. Stop Smoking Intervention and Services. NICE guideline (2014) https://www.nice.org.uk/guidance/ng92, accessed 7 Nov. 2021.

# CHAPTER 8
# Obesity and Diabetes (Diabesity)

Issues like obesity do, as you well know, have a knock-on effect to diabetes.
So, we all are better off if we invest early in prevention.
**Jacinda Ardern**

## Epidemiology of Obesity

According to the WHO, obesity reached epidemic proportions globally by 2014. More than 1 billion people are overweight, with 300 million of them obese. [1] (**Figure 8.1**) Obesity is generally centred in the developed countries. The Organisation of Economic Cooperation and Development (OECD) has estimated that obesity and overweight are rising at the rate of 67% among the US population. Further, it is estimated that, by 2025, three-quarters of the US population will be obese. [2]

Obesity in the United Kingdom has trebled in the last thirty years, and it's expected that more than half of the population will be obese by 2050.[2] It has the second highest level of obesity behind Hungary in Europe and is, therefore, dubbed the 'fat man of Europe'. [3] Obesity epidemic in the developing world is rising at an alarming rate as well. The Asian region is now the epicentre of obesity, with millions in India and China are obese. The Pacific region is seeing one of the highest obesity epidemics in the world. Countries like Nauru, Tonga, Samoa, Fiji, Cook Islands, and Papua New Guinea have high prevalence of obesity. [4] More females than males are affected in this epidemic, and childhood obesity is also in epidemic proportion.

The obesity epidemic is, therefore, on both a regional and global scale. Obesity poses significant risks for cardiovascular diseases, diabetes, hypertension, stroke, and certain cancers.

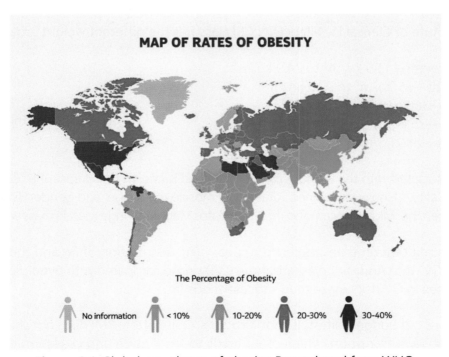

**Figure 8.1.** Global prevalence of obesity. Reproduced from WHO.

**The obesity epidemic is global. While the highest numbers of obesity are found in the developed world, the numbers are rising in the developing world, with Asia Pacific being among the epicentres of the global obesity pandemic.**

## Diagnostic Tools for Obesity

There are several measures of obesity currently in use, and they can be classified under two groups—the field methods and the reference measurement methods.

### Field Methods

Body mass index (BMI) is the easiest method in the category of field methods, among others such as the waist circumference, waist-to-hip ratio, skin folds thickness, and bioelectrical impedance. The field methods are extensively used in clinics and for research purposes because they are simple and easy to use. These methods include:

- Body mass index
- Waist circumference
- Waist-to-hip ratio
- Skin fold thickness
- Bioelectrical impedance

Body Mass Index (BMI)

BMI is the ratio of a person's weight in kilograms to his/her height in metres squared ($kg/m^2$). It is a simple, efficient, and effective way to classify a person's weight and is used as a screening tool for diagnosing overweight/obesity.

The National Institute of Clinical Excellence (NICE) classifies the different weight groups as follows: [5]

- Healthy weight—18.5 $kg/m^2$ to 24.9 $kg/m^2$
- Overweight—25 $kg/m^2$ to 29.9 $kg/m^2$
- Obesity I—30 $kg/m^2$ to 34.9 $kg/m^2$
- Obesity II—35 $kg/m^2$ to 39.9 $kg/m^2$
- Obesity III—≥40 $kg/m^2$

BMI is strongly associated with the amount of body fats and is known to increase the risks of cardiovascular diseases and mortality. [6] However, it is not adjusted to muscle mass, age, and gender. Therefore, it does not differentiate between the 'Michelin Man' and the 'Terminator Man' with huge muscle mass who has a higher BMI.

Further, BMI does not differentiate 'apples from peas'. The distribution of fat and the location of the fat mass determines CV risks. Android obesity is more CVD prone compared with gynoid obesity, and visceral obesity predisposes to CV risks more than subcutaneous fat. [7]

Moreover, BMI does not budge in lifestyle modifications. Quite often, BMI does not change when patients embark on a lifestyle prescription, which often leads to frustration and cessation of the prescription. Healthcare workers need to be prepared to help patients who experience this situation.

## Waist Circumference

Waist circumference is another method of measuring a person's obesity. The accurate position for measuring the waist circumference is midway between the uppermost border of iliac crest and lower border of the rib cage. The tape has to be placed around the abdomen at the level of the midpoint, and the reading should be taken when the tape is snug and not compressing the skin. In very overweight patients, it may be difficult to accurately palpate the bony landmarks, so placing the tape at the level of the belly button is recommended in practice.

The International Diabetes Association gives cut-off waist circumferences at:

- ≥94 cm for Caucasian men
- ≥80 cm for Caucasian women
- ≥90 cm for Asian men (based on Chinese/Malay)
- ≥80 cm for Asian women (based on Chinese/Malay)

Waist circumference is the easiest and least expensive method of measuring body fats, and it has a very good correlation with accurate methods, such as the CT and MRI. Waist circumference is the best anthropometric predictor of visceral fat. [8] It seems to be a stronger independent predictor of cardiovascular disease than the BMI. [9-10]

However, there are no standardised ranges for all ethnicities. [11] Asians have a lower waist circumference because of more visceral fat content that predisposes to CV diseases.

## Waist-to-Hip Ratio

The waist-to-hip ratio is another way of assessing the abdominal obesity, where the waist measurement is divided by the hip measurement in centimetres. In women it is expected be ≤0.8, and in men, the expectation is ≤1. (This means that, in women, the waist should be narrower than the hips, and in men, the waist should be narrower or the same as the hips.) Waist-to-hip ratio is useful in smaller people whose waist circumference alone can underestimate their obesity risks.

A study has shown that waist-to-hip ratio correlates with the complications of obesity. [12]

## Skin Fold Thickness

The skin fold thickness measurement is another method of measuring obesity. There are three to nine different sites in the body where this assessment can be done, but the right side of the body is usually used for the purpose of consistency.

It is an uncomfortable test, where the tester pinches the test site, creating a double layer—the adipose tissue layer below and the skin above. The calliper is then applied at a right angle at 1 cm at the lower layer, and the thickness is measured in two seconds. The mean of two readings is taken, but if they're different than a third reading is taken, and the median is finally taken as the skin fold thickness. [13]

A study published in the *American Journal of Nutrition* showed that the skin fold measurement tended to underestimate body fat calculation compared with underwater weighing and total body mass assessments. This was due to the technical difficulty in not being able to have a large enough sample size due to fewer callipers being available.[3]

Skin fold thickness is not a robust method in measuring childhood obesity. Therefore, it should be used as an index and not a measure of obesity in this population until it is validated by further studies in this population. Previous studies looking into this tool have had wide variations and published equations have errors.[4]

## Reference Measurement Methods

Reference measurement methods are more sophisticated techniques used in research settings to validate body measurement. Although they are more accurate than the field methods, they are rarely used in the clinical settings due to their high costs and the fact that the field techniques are easy and cost-effective. They include:

- Computed tomography (CT)
- Magnetic resonance imaging (MRI)
- Dual X-ray absorptiometry (DEXA)

Computed Tomography (CT) / Magnetic Resonance Imaging (MRI)

The gold standard for the quantitative assessment of intra-abdominal adipose tissue is CT and MRI.[5] With their excellent resolutions of adipose tissue, CT and MRI are direct method of assessing visceral fat deposition in both adult and paediatric populations. They are accurate and allow for measurements of specific body fats, such as percutaneous and visceral fats. However, they are expensive, immobile, and cannot accommodate certain patient populations, such as pregnant women, children, obese patients, and those with devices implantations like older types of pacemakers and CRTs in heart failure patients.

These techniques of measuring body fats, for now, remain merely research tools and not for clinical use.

### Measures of Obesity

1. Field methods
   - BMI
   - Waist circumference
   - Waist-to-hip ratio
   - Skin Fold

2. Reference measurement methods
   - Computed tomography (CT)
   - Magnetic resonance imaging (MRI)
   - Dual X-ray absorptiometry (DEXA)

## Pathophysiology of Obesity

Obesity is characterised by the storages of excessive fatty tissues in the body. Subcutaneous fatty tissues can be visible in the abdomen (android obesity), often called the 'apple-shaped' in men and around the pelvis (gynoid obesity), often called the 'pear-shaped'. The most deadly and innocuous fatty tissues are the visceral fats.

Obesity is a by-product of multiple contributing factors from the environment and the genes. Therefore, it has truly a 'polygenic' etiology.

### Environmental Contribution

Storage of fat in the human body is a survival mechanism in times of fasting and starvation. However, the current obesity epidemic is predominantly secondary to the changes in lifestyle in an 'obesogenic environment'. Lack of exercise, access to cars, long hours of television, and access to high carbohydrate and fatty diets are universal contributors of obesity epidemic. In addition, cultural and religious perceptions play significant roles in fuelling the epidemic. For example, obesity is deemed as healthy and is associated with an affluent life in some parts of the world.

### Genetic Contribution

Monogenic disease (5% obesity)

Several genes are already known to predispose individuals who acquired those genes to develop obesity. These obesities are categorically termed the monogenic or syndromic obesity or pure forms of obesity. The ob gene in mice and the leptin gene in humans [17] set the precedence for further research into obesity genetics, which revealed more genes associated with appetite regulation. [18]

Some examples of monogenetic obesities are Prader Willi syndrome in males and the Angelman syndrome in females, along with the Moon Bardet-Biedl syndrome, which is associated with mental retardation and other systemic abnormalities. These genetic conditions contribute to only 5% of the obesity prevalence.

*Polygenic Disease*

Several genes are known to be associated with obesity. [19] However, these genes are not 'destiny genes,' [20] meaning many people who carry these genes do not become obese and that other factors from the environment influence the phenotype. [6]

---

- **95% of all obesity is polygenic caused by environmental factors and 'non-destiny genes'**
- **5% of all obesity is monogenic caused by 'destiny genes'**

---

## Types of Fat Distribution and Impacts on Lifestyle Diseases

There are two types of fats based on their anatomical locations and their propensities to cause associated comorbidities. They are only differentiated by MRI and they are:

- Visceral fat
- Subcutaneous fat

### Visceral Fat

Visceral fat is body fat stored within the abdominal cavity, around important internal organs such as the liver, pancreas, and intestines. It is referred to as the 'active fat', since increased visceral fat is associated with insulin resistance leading to type 2 diabetes, breast cancer, colorectal cancer, heart disease, and Alzheimer's.

## Subcutaneous Adipose Tissue (SAT)

Subcutaneous fat lies right beneath the skin and is called subcutaneous adipose tissue (SAT) and measured by the help of skin fold callipers to assess total body fat. It is divided into two types by the fascial plane and tends to have distinctive contributions to the complications of obesity:

- superficial SAT (sSAT)
- deep SAT (dSAT).

*Superficial Subcutaneous Adipose Tissue (sSAT)*

The sSAT has less lipolysis, lipogenesis, inflammation, and risk of insulin resistance than the dSAT. Therefore, it is less harmful and behaves like the SAT of the lower body in the hips, thighs, and buttocks

*Deep Subcutaneous Adipose Tissue (dSAT)*

The dSAT is mostly located in the posterior half of the abdomen. It is the most active component of the SAT, where the rate of processes like lipolysis, lipogenesis, and inflammatory protein expression is higher than in the sSAT. [21] The complications of the dSAT have been shown to be closely relate to the pathophysiology of obesity complications of VAT (visceral adipose tissue). The sSAT, however, is less active and, therefore, tends to follow the less pathogenic pattern of the lower-body SAT. [22]

A large abdomen can be the result of an increase in both types of fat.

### Types of Fat Distribution

1. Visceral
2. Subcutaneous
   - superficial SAT (sSAT)
   - deep SAT (dSAT)

# Gender and Ethnic Variations of Adipose Tissues[7]

## Gender Variation of Adiposity

CT and the MRI techniques have contributed to identifying gender and racial differences in body compositions, including patterns of body composition changes during weight loss.

Females have more total fat (adipose tissue), with a large quantity in the lower trunk and the pelvic region that contributes to gynoid obesity, often colloquially called 'pear-shaped obesity'. They have less total muscle (lean tissue) than males. Women in their twenties and thirties are less likely to be obese, but in menopause, they have increased VAT.

Males have more visceral and hepatic adiposity, with concentration around the abdomen that contributes to android obesity, colloquially known as the 'apple-shaped obesity', which increases the risks of insulin resistance, CAD, cancers, and other health issues.

- **Android obesity in men predisposes them to insulin resistance, CAD, and some forms of cancers.**
- **Gynoid obesity in women has less predisposition to insulin resistance, CAD, and cancers.**

### Racial and Ethnic Variation in Adiposity

It was observed using CT scans that lean Japanese American males with low BMI had increased VAT and insulin resistance. Asian American females have a higher VAT proportion compared to Caucasian females. Although African American females have less VAT and more upper body subcutaneous adipose tissue SAT, their upper body obesity is not associated with increased mortality as seen in Caucasian women.

Pacific women have high lower-body obesity and are less prone to CAD, insulin resistance, and cancers.

Visceral fats vary in gender and ethnicities, which potentially explains the differences in CAD seen in various groups throughout the world. Caucasians, African American men, and Indian women seem to have more visceral fats.

## The Roles of Adipose Tissues

Visceral adipose tissue functions as an endocrine organ and is involved in a complex interplay between inflammation and obesity-related complications. It secretes adipokines, such as interleukin (IL)-6, tumour necrosis factor-α (TNF-α), macrophage chemoattractant protein-1 (MCP-1), and resistin, which induce insulin resistance and vascular endothelial dysfunction leading to CAD. On the other hand, visceral fat might have beneficial metabolic effects by producing adiponectin, which increases insulin sensitivity and decreases glucose intolerance and diabetes. However, the evidence for this is weak and more research is needed.[8]

### Complications of Obesity

Obesity is associated with many complications, including social, medical, and financial complications. Social complications include stigmatisation and social discourse. The myriad of medical complications ultimately leads to ill health. These result in both high direct and high indirect financial costs to patients and their families and to the healthcare systems.

The medical complications of obesity can be classified into two types:

- Metabolic
- Non-Metabolic

Metabolic Complications

Metabolic complications of obesity include:

- Insulin resistance
- Hyperinsulinaemia
- Diabetes
- Dyslipidaemia

### Non-Metabolic Complications

Non-metabolic complications of obesity include:

- Cardiovascular diseases
- Non-alcoholic steatohepatitis, pancreatitis, and cholelithiasis
- Pickwickian syndrome
- Cancers such as breast, oesophagus, colon, endometrium, and renal
- Osteoarthritis
- Polycystic ovarian syndrome

*Obesity Hypoventilation Syndrome (Pickwickian Syndrome)*

Pickwickian, or obesity hypoventilation syndrome as it is known clinically, is a respiratory complication of obesity seen in some obese patients. It is associated with obstructive sleep apnoea caused by upper airway obstruction due to flail glottis blocking the trachea during sleep. Ventilatory centres in the brainstem tend to have a lower drive than in those who do not have this syndrome. This results in hypoxemia from hypoventilation associated with hypercapnia. Pulmonary hypertension and heart failure is ensured if left untreated.

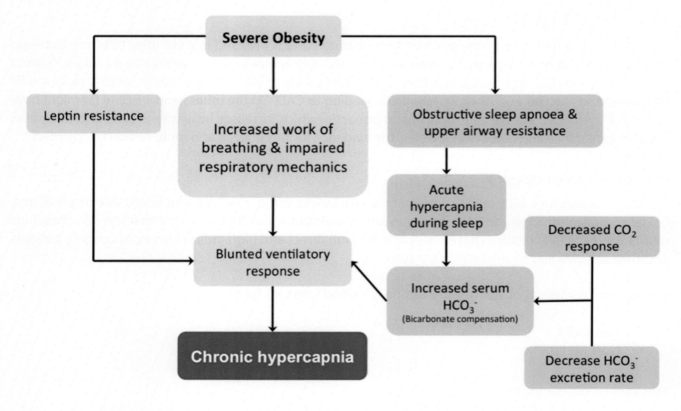

**Figure 8.2** Mechanism of Pickwickian Syndrome. Reproduced from Mokhlesi B. (2010). Obesity hypoventilation syndrome: a state-of-the-art review. Respiratory care, 55(10), 1347–1365.

### The Role of Adipose Tissues in the Pathogenesis of Diabetes

'Diabesity' is a term coined to describe the concomitant occurrence of obesity and diabetes. Although, these two conditions are interdependent, it is difficult to explain their association. Among many other theories proposed as the causes of obesity-related complications, two theories stand out in their possible contributions to insulin resistance and other complications:

- Portal theory
- Inflammatory theory

**Portal Theory**

This theory highlights that the high free fatty acid (FFA) discharged into the portal vein noted among obese individuals is associated with hepatic insulin resistance and steatosis. [9, 25]

Other studies, however, show that the FFA from the visceral fat is minimal and could contribute less to the pathogenesis of insulin resistance. [26, 27]

**Inflammatory Theory**

Visceral fats also increase secretion of inflammatory adipokines into the portal vein, which sustains a low level of persistent inflammation in the vasculature. These adipokines include interleukin (IL)-6, tumour necrosis factor-α (TNF-α), macrophage chemoattractant protein-1 (MCP-1), resistin, and retinol binding protein 4 (RBP4), which are thought to induce insulin resistance and diabetes more than the free fatty acids. Therefore, cytokines are proposed to be contributing more significantly to the insulin resistance than FFA.

| *Two Theories Explaining Obesity-Related Complications* |
| --- |
| 1. Inflammatory theory—more potent<br>2. Portal theory—less potent |

## Role of Obesity in Cancers

Whilst the mechanisms by which obesity either causes and/or is associated with cancers are not fully understood, there is a strong association of obesity with hormone sensitive cancers such as breast, endometrium, and prostate cancers. Others that are strongly linked to cancer, according to the International Agency for Research on Cancer (IARC), are colon, oesophageal, adenocarcinoma, renal cell carcinoma, ovarian, and pancreas. **Figure 8.3** shows possible mechanisms in obesity leading to cancer. Further, obesity is also associated with increased deaths in cancers. The relative risks of dying from established cancers among obese patients increases 1.5 and 1.6 folds in men and women respectively. [28]

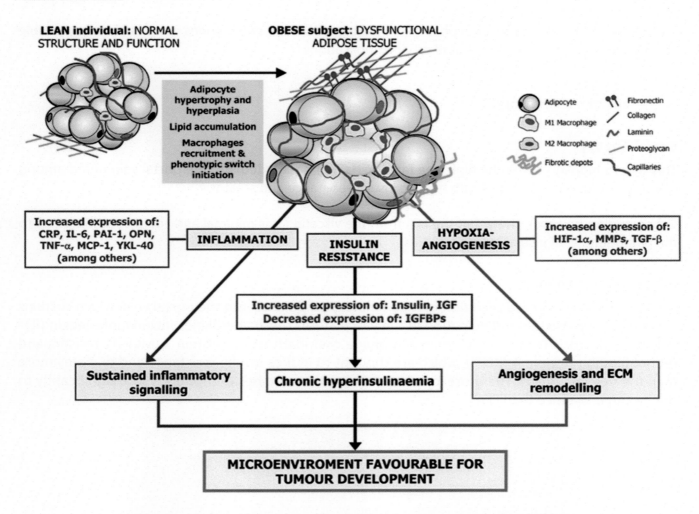

**Figure 8.3** Possible cancer-causing mechanisms in obesity. Reproduced from Hernandez et al., 'Mechanisms Linking Excess Adiposity with Carcinogenesis Promotion', *Frontiers in Endocrinology*, 2014 (2014), 00065.

# Management of Obesity

## Tiered Level of Obesity Management

A classical tiered level of addressing the obesity epidemic has been initiated by the Welsh government called the Wales Obesity Pathway. This pathway has four levels at which obesity can be managed.

Level 1: Community-Based Early Intervention and Prevention

The communities are empowered several approaches: through education about the dietary approaches, provision of exercise spaces for exercises, lifestyle education in schools and provision of the basic healthcare at the community level .

Level 2: Community and Primary Weight Management Programmes

The community provides various weight-losing programmes for its members and conducts health check programmes to identify obese members and facilitate interventions.

Level 3: Specialists Multidisciplinary Weight Management Services

Services that specialise in dieting, exercise, behavioural, and pharmacological interventions to prevent and address obesity are offered.

Level 4: Specialists Medical and Surgical Services

Pharmacotherapy and bariatric surgery services in addressing obesity are explored at this level.

## Lifestyle modifications

### Dietary Prescription

Dietary prescription is the standard and first line in obesity management. It can be prescribed based on several factors, which any prescriber must consider:

- Presence or absence of comorbidities
- Food availability
- Patient preferences
- Religious and cultural beliefs

Different dietary regimens are used in the management of obesity. However, the essential principle of weight-losing diet is based on the principle of 'less intake and more output', where the energy balance is tipped towards negativity. These can be achieved with intake of fewer carbohydrates, fewer fats, and more vegetables.

Diabetes prevention studies have shown that dietary prescription alone does not lead to significant weight loss. In fact, both diet and exercise tend to have positive impact on weight loss and diabetes. Application of this principle in obesity management is reasonable.

### Exercises Prescription

Weight loss is a long-term effect of exercise. The primary diabetes prevention studies have demonstrated that supervised exercise regimens, both aerobic and resistance exercises, were better in not only preventing and remitting diabetes but also in reducing weight. The HART-D Trial further consolidated this by providing more evidence that, when you combine aerobic exercise with resistance training, there is reduction in belly fat, reduction in waistline, and improved functional capacity, which lowers glucose. [29] These findings are consistent with the current recommendations.

### Multidisciplinary Management (MDT)

Like all other chronic diseases, good management of obesity requires a committed patient with expert MDT management to achieve optimal outcomes. [30, 31] The MDT approach includes behavioural change therapists.

## Pharmacotherapy

There were many anti-obesity drugs that were trialled but were withdrawn by the FDA for various reasons, including safety and efficacy issues. The following sections will discuss a variety of these drugs for academic purposes.

## Sibutramine

Sibutramine is a combined norepinephrine and serotonin reuptake inhibitor the FDA approved in 1997 for BMI ≥27 kg/m² with other comorbidities or for ≥30 kg/m². It was withdrawn three years later in 2010 in the United States and Europe because of increased cardiovascular events.

## Rimonabant

This anorexigenic (anti-appetite) anti-obesity drug acts through the cannabinoid receptor CB1 by reducing appetite. Although, the benefits of improving cardiometabolic profile spread across all CV risk factors, the risk of serious psychiatric complications, including suicide, was serious, warranting withdrawal by the European Medicine Agency in January 2010. It was not approved by the FDA.

## Phentermine/Topiramate (Qsymia)

This drug combination increases the release of epinephrine in the hypothalamus, causing appetite suppression. Its safety effects are not known. EMA rejected the drug in February 2013.

## Lorcaserin

Lorcaserin is a serotogenic anti-obesity drug. It has serotonergic actions, causing appetite suppression and was approved by the FDA in June 2012 for treating obesity, with a lot of scepticism, given its delays and multiple reviews with the FDA. [32]

## Orlistat

Orlistat is the only anti-obesity drug currently in use. It works by inhibiting gastric and pancreatic lipases, which breaks down fats for digestion. Thus, it prevents around a third of the ingested fat from absorption . This undigested fat is not absorbed and is passed out with faeces. This can cause loose and greasy steatorrhea stool.

This helps reduce weight gain but won't necessarily cause one to lose weight. Therefore, it's still important to follow a recommended diet and exercise plan.

Orlistat is only recommended if an individual has made significant effort to lose weight through diet, exercise, or lifestyle changes and has:

- BMI of ≥28 kg/m² or more and other obesity related conditions, such as high blood pressure, dyslipidaemia, diabetes, and cardiovascular diseases
- a BMI of ≥30 kg/m²

Treatment with orlistat should only continue beyond three months if an individual has lost 5% of his or her body weight. Physicians/GPs must carry out a review by end of this period and determine the continuity of orlistat.

Studies have shown that, on average, orlistat plus a weight-reducing diet and exercise causes more weight loss than a weight-reducing diet and exercise alone. Some people lose 10% or more of their body weight within six months with the help of orlistat. In others, it is less effective.

## Liraglutide

NICE has recently approved liraglutide, a once-daily GLP-1 analogue injection, for managing obesity alongside a calorie-controlled diet and increased physical activity. The trial data for liraglutide shows a more modest but significant effect on weight loss (-4.32% weight relative to placebo over a three-year period). Importantly, it also delays the development of type 2 diabetes and reduces CVS disease. [33]

NICE has, therefore, set the following criteria for use of liraglutide in obesity:

- BMI >35 (or >32.5 if from a minority ethnic group at higher risk of complications of obesity) *and*
- Presence of non-diabetic hyperglycaemia (in other words, prediabetes) *and*
- At high risk of cardiovascular disease based on risk factors (for example, hypertension and dyslipidaemia)

| *Two Approved Anti-Obesity Drugs Currently in Clinical Use* |
|---|
| 1. Orlistat<br>2. Liraglutide |

## Bariatric Surgery

Bariatric (anti-obesity) surgery is one of the treatment modalities of obesity. It has been shown to treat obesity and also improve the obese patients' metabolic profile and remits [34, 35] and prevent the development of diabetes.[36] Furthermore, it reduces cardiovascular and cancer mortalities. [37-39]

Although, diabetes remission rates are quite good in this surgery, with improved metabolic profile, the complications are real and serious. Some patients undergo revision surgery that puts them at even higher risk, an area that does not have good robust evidence. Therefore, for bariatric surgery to be successful, strict criteria must be met, a risk-benefit analysis must be done, and patients must make an informed decision on the type of surgery.

Bariatric surgery, therefore, could serve only a few of the patients who meet these requirements and should not be seen as the answer to the obesity epidemic.

## Types of Anti-Obesity Surgery

There are different types of anti-obesity surgeries, and these are carried out according to the patients' choices. It is beyond the remit of this book to discuss these types; however, for simplicity, they are classified under three main categories based on the mechanisms:

- Restrictive bariatric surgery
- Malabsorptive bariatric surgery
- Mixed procedures

> **Three Mechanisms of Bariatric Surgeries**
>
> 1. Restrictive
> 2. Malabsorptive
> 3. Mixed

The two most widely used procedures to achieve restriction and malabsorption, and or both are: [40]

1. Gastric banding—based on restriction of stomach space
2. Gastric Bypass—based on restriction and malabsorption

| Features | Bypass | Banding |
|---|---|---|
| Technically | Demanding | Less demanding |
| Weight Loss | More weight loss (2/3 of weight) | Less weight loss (½ Weight loss) |
| Complications | High risk of complications and death (1 in 5) | Low risk of complications (1 in 10) |
| Reversibility | No | Yes |
| Method of surgery | Endoscopic | Endoscopic |

**Table 8.1** Comparisons between the two widely used bariatric surgeries.

Other less commonly used bariatric surgical procedures are:

1. Sleeve gastrectomy
   This is used in patients with BMI of $\geq 60$ kg/m² for whom bypass and banding pose potential high risks. It is used as a bridge method before bypass or banding is done when the patient loses 60 to 70% of his or her body weight. It involves surgical removal of three-quarters of the stomach.

2. Biliopancreatic diversion
   This procedure is similar to a bypass, except that it involves a larger bypass of the small intestine, leading to less absorption. It has a good outcome, with 80% expected weight loss but has more complications and unpleasant diarrhoea than other bariatric procedures. It is recommended when rapid weight loss is required to prevent serious complications from causing the rapid deterioration of health.

3. Intra-gastric balloon
   This is a temporary procedure, and the balloon is removed after six months in patients who don't meet the criteria but are obese. A soft silicon balloon is inserted into the stomach to reduce stomach size. The balloon is filled with air or water to regulate the size of the stomach, and the procedure I is done endoscopically, rather than by bypass.

## Indications for Bariatric Surgery

NICE's old guidelines indicate that bariatric surgery in obese individuals must be employed as a last resort in those who:

- Are classified as having class III obesity (BMI >40 kg/m2)
- Are classified as having class II obesity (BMI 35–39 kg/m2) in the presence of comorbidities and inability to achieve weight-loss maintenance following adequate trial of health behaviour interventions and anti-obesity pharmacotherapy with orlistat
- Agree to lifelong follow-up at an obesity clinic after surgery

There is no evidence comparing lifestyle modifications, pharmacotherapy, and bariatric surgery. That is why NICE recommends bariatric surgery only in patients who have tried other treatment modalities and have failed and accept to be followed up post bariatric surgery.

## Mechanisms of Weight Loss after Bariatric (Anti-Obesity) Surgery

Hormonal changes after the bariatric surgery underline the mechanisms of weight loss, prevention, and remission of diabetes and even changes in the metabolic profile.

GLP-1 and Peptide YY are released in large amounts after bypass surgery. Both decrease appetite, resulting in weight loss in a few days after surgery.

Ghrelin is an appetite stimulant hormone (hunger hormone) released from the stomach and is in high concentration in obese patients. However, in those with gastric bypass, the ghrelin hormone is low, and so leptin (satiety hormone) level rises. This rise in leptin, among other effects, further reduces ghrelin, leading to low food intake.

---

- **Bariatric surgery increases the satiety hormone leptin, GLP1 RA, and peptide YY and reduces ghrelin—the appetite stimulant hormone.**
- **These changes cause a net effect of reducing appetite and increasing weight loss.**

---

## Complications of Bariatric Surgery

There are different classifications of complications of bariatric surgery. For example, complications may be classed according to time after surgery (acute versus chronic complications) or may be categorised related to anaesthetic complications, such as perioperative, operative, and post-operative.

Essentially, the complications are dependent on the *type of bariatric surgery* a patient decides to receive, with appropriate information given by the managing team of surgeons and dietitians. It is beyond the remit of this book to explain the varied complications of each type of bariatric procedure. The reader is advised to seek appropriate textbooks for further clarifications.

## The Effects of Bariatric Surgery on Type 2 Diabetes Mellitus

Bariatric surgery can induce a sustainably improved glycaemic control of T2DM and other comorbidities in severely obese patients. The change in glycaemic control is seen in days, even before weight loss is noted.

There are no RCTs done so far to confirm the beneficial effect of bariatric surgery on diabetes. However, what is available is from general non-randomised observational studies, indicating improved glycaemic control, increased insulin sensitivity, remission of diabetes post-surgery, and improved quality of life. For example, the Greenville observation showed that 82.9% of the 165 patients with T2DM remained in remission after the roux-en-Y gastric bypass. [41] This was, however, an uncontrolled surgical case series.

The Swedish Obese Study (SOS Study) had 156 obese diabetic patients divided into two arms (bariatric surgery and control). This study showed that the number requiring no drug to maintain remission doubled in the surgical arm as compared to the control.[42]

Several small studies have confirmed these observations in Greenville and SOS. Bariatric surgery has favourable effects on other CV risk factors. However, there are no data on the long-term effect of bariatric surgery on the progression of microvascular complications or cost-effectiveness as compared with other available therapies of diabetes treatment.

Bariatric surgery is the last resort for those who have unsuccessfully tried lifestyle modifications with anti-obesity pharmacotherapy. The criteria for this procedure are quite strict, and therefore, not all severely obese patients with or without diabetes will require bariatric surgery. For these reasons, bariatric surgery is not an answer to the obesity epidemic.

## Effect of Bariatric Surgery on Type 1 Obese Diabetes Mellitus

Patients with T1DM mediated by idiopathic insulinopenia and the immune mediated are generally thin or have normal weights. Those with ketosis prone T1DM that simulates T2DM can have obesity with poor glycaemic control. A case report suggests that bariatric surgery can potentially improve metabolic and glycaemic control in this group.[43]

---

- **Bariatric surgery is only indicated for those who have failed to lose weight with physical and pharmacological interventions and agree to lifelong follow-up after the surgery.**
- **Bariatric surgery is not an answer to the obesity epidemic—not least because it has serious complications.**
- **However, bariatric surgery improves metabolic profile of severely obese patients, including glycaemic control in those with both T1DM and T2DM.**

---

## Key Messages:

- **Obesity has been at epidemic level globally, with the majority in the developed world. The epicentre has now shifted to the Asia Pacific region with a high prevalence in India and China.**
- **Field methods are commonly used to assess obesity.**
- **Obesity is predominantly polygenic caused by both the environment and the genetic predisposition.**
- **Visceral fats predispose people to complications of obesity like diabetes, through either the process of releasing inflammatory markers and/or an increase in the release of FFA.**
- **The dSAT contributes proportionately to the complications of obesity.**
- **The sSAT and gynoid obesity do not contribute to cardiovascular disease and diabetes.**
- **Management of obesity on a tiered level community-based anti-obesity service could include lifestyle changes, pharmacotherapy, and even escalation to anti-obesity surgery for those meeting the criteria.**

## References

1   Obesity and Overweight. WHO Fact Sheet. https://www. fact sheet_02 (who.int)

2   Obesity Update (2017). OECD. https://www. Obesity-Update-2017.pdf (oecd.org)

3   Obesity Crisis. The Daily Mail Online. https://www. Obesity crisis has turned the UK into the fat man of Europe | Daily Mail Online

4   Pacific Islanders pay heavy price for abandoning traditional diet. WHO Bulletin. https://www. WHO | Pacific islanders pay heavy price for abandoning traditional diet

5   Obesity, Identification, Assessment and Management. NICE Clinical Guideline CG189. https://www.nice.org.uk/guidance/cg189

6   Calle, E. E., Thun, M. J., Petrelli, J. M., Rodriguez, C., & Heath, C. W., Jr (1999). Body-mass index and mortality in a prospective cohort of U.S. adults. *The New England journal of medicine*, *341*(15), 1097–1105. https://doi.org/10.1056/NEJM199910073411501

7   Why BMI is a Poor Measure of Your Health. http://blogs.plos.org/obesitypanacea/2012/02/10/why-the-body-mass-index-bmi-is-a-poor-measure-of-your-health/

8   Han, T. S., van Leer, E. M., Seidell, J. C., & Lean, M. E. (1996). Waist circumference as a screening tool for cardiovascular risk factors: evaluation of receiver operating characteristics (ROC). *Obesity research*, *4*(6), 533–547. https://doi.org/10.1002/j.1550-8528.1996.tb00267.x

9   Balkau, B., Deanfield, J. E., Després, J. P.,et.al., (2007). International Day for the Evaluation of Abdominal Obesity (IDEA): a study of waist circumference, cardiovascular disease, and diabetes mellitus in 168,000 primary care patients in 63 countries. *Circulation*, *116*(17), 1942–1951. https://doi.org/10.1161/CIRCULATIONAHA.106.676379

10  Waist circumference and Cardiometabolic Risk. https://www.care.diabetesjournals.org/content/30/6/1647.full

11  From Calipers to Scans. Ten ways of telling whether the body is Fat or Lean. http://www.hsph.harvard.edu/obesity-prevention-source/obesity-definition/how-to-measure-body-fatness/

12  Tran, N., Blizzard, C. L., Luong, K. N., et.al.,(2018). The importance of waist circumference and body mass index in cross-sectional relationships with risk of cardiovascular disease in Vietnam. *PloS one*, *13*(5), e0198202. https://doi.org/10.1371/journal.pone.0198202

13  Skin Fold Measurement. http://www.topendsports.com/testing/skinfold-sites.htm.

14  Skin Fold thickness in obese subjects. http://ajcn.nutrition.org/content/51/4/571.full.pdf+html

15  Reilly, J. J., Wilson, J., & Durnin, J. V. (1995). Determination of body composition from skinfold thickness: a validation study. *Archives of disease in childhood*, *73*(4), 305–310. https://doi.org/10.1136/adc.73.4.305

16  Shuster, A., Patlas, M., Pinthus, J. H., & Mourtzakis, M. (2012). The clinical importance of visceral adiposity: a critical review of methods for visceral adipose tissue analysis. *The British journal of radiology*, *85*(1009), 1–10. https://doi.org/10.1259/bjr/38447238

17  Zhang, Y., Proenca, R., Maffei, M.,et.al.,(1994). Positional cloning of the mouse obese gene and its human homologue. *Nature*, *372*(6505), 425–432. https://doi.org/10.1038/372425a0

18  Montague, C. T., Farooqi, I. S., Whitehead, J. P.,et.al., (1997). Congenital leptin deficiency is associated with severe early-onset obesity in humans. *Nature*, *387*(6636), 903–908. https://doi.org/10.1038/43185

19  Rankinen, T., Zuberi, A., Chagnon, Y. C., et.al., (2006). The human obesity gene map: the 2005 update. *Obesity (Silver Spring, Md.), 14*(4), 529–644. https://doi.org/10.1038/oby.2006.71

20  *Genes are not Destiny. https//*www.hsph.harvard.edu/obesity-prevention.../obesity.../genes-and-obesity

21  Cancello, R., Zulian, A., Gentilini, D.,et.al.,(2013). Molecular and morphologic characterization of superficial- and deep-subcutaneous adipose tissue subdivisions in human obesity. *Obesity (Silver Spring, Md.), 21*(12), 2562–2570. https://doi.org/10.1002/oby.20417

22  Golan, R., Shelef, I., Rudich, A.,et.al.,(2012). Abdominal superficial subcutaneous fat: a putative distinct protective fat subdepot in type 2 diabetes. *Diabetes care, 35*(3), 640–647. https://doi.org/10.2337/dc11-1583

23  Silver, H. J., Welch, E. B., Avison, M. J., & Niswender, K. D. (2010). Imaging body composition in obesity and weight loss: challenges and opportunities. *Diabetes, metabolic syndrome and obesity : targets and therapy, 3,* 337–347. https://doi.org/10.2147/DMSOTT.S9454

24  Fontana, L., Eagon, J. C., Trujillo, M. E.,et.al.,(2007). Visceral fat adipokine secretion is associated with systemic inflammation in obese humans. *Diabetes, 56*(4), 1010–1013. https://doi.org/10.2337/db06-1656

25  Després, J. P., Moorjani, S., Lupien, P. J.,et.al.,(1990). Regional distribution of body fat, plasma lipoproteins, and cardiovascular disease. *Arteriosclerosis (Dallas, Tex.), 10*(4), 497–511. https://doi.org/10.1161/01.atv.10.4.497

26  Boden G. (1997). Role of fatty acids in the pathogenesis of insulin resistance and NIDDM. *Diabetes, 46*(1), 3–10.

27  Nielsen, S., Guo, Z., Johnson, C. M.,et.al., (2004). Splanchnic lipolysis in human obesity. *The Journal of clinical investigation, 113*(11), 1582–1588. https://doi.org/10.1172/JCI21047

28  Klein S. (2004). The case of visceral fat: argument for the defense. *The Journal of clinical investigation, 113*(11), 1530–1532. https://doi.org/10.1172/JCI22028

29  Malnick, S. D., & Knobler, H. (2006). The medical complications of obesity. *QJM : monthly journal of the Association of Physicians, 99*(9), 565–579. https://doi.org/10.1093/qjmed/hcl085

30  Church, T. S., Blair, S. N., Cocreham, S., et.al.,(2010). Effects of aerobic and resistance training on hemoglobin A1c levels in patients with type 2 diabetes: a randomized controlled trial. *JAMA, 304*(20), 2253–2262. https://doi.org/10.1001/jama.2010.1710

31  Dennis, E. A., Dengo, A. L., Comber, D. L.,et.al.,(2010). Water consumption increases weight loss during a hypocaloric diet intervention in middle-aged and older adults. *Obesity (Silver Spring, Md.), 18*(2), 300–307. https://doi.org/10.1038/oby.2009.235

32  Dubnov-Raz, G., Constantini, N. W., Yariv, H., et.al.,(2011). Influence of water drinking on resting energy expenditure in overweight children. *International journal of obesity (2005), 35*(10), 1295–1300. https://doi.org/10.1038/ijo.2011.130

33  Smith, S. R., Weissman, N. J., Anderson, C. M.,et.al., & Behavioral Modification and Lorcaserin for Overweight and Obesity Management (BLOOM) Study Group (2010). Multicenter, placebo-controlled trial of lorcaserin for weight management. *The New England journal of medicine, 363*(3), 245–256. https://doi.org/10.1056/NEJMoa0909809

34  le Roux, C. W., Astrup, A., Fujioka, K.,et.al.,& SCALE Obesity Prediabetes NN8022-1839 Study Group (2017). 3 years of liraglutide versus placebo for type 2 diabetes risk reduction and weight management in individuals with prediabetes: a randomised, double-blind trial. *Lancet (London, England), 389*(10077), 1399–1409. https://doi.org/10.1016/S0140-6736(17)30069-7

35  Brethauer, S. A., Aminian, A., Romero-Talamás, et.al.,(2013). Can diabetes be surgically cured? Long-term metabolic effects of bariatric surgery in obese patients with type 2 diabetes mellitus. *Annals of surgery, 258*(4), 628–637. https://doi.org/10.1097/SLA.0b013e3182a5034b

36  Adams, T. D., Davidson, L. E., Litwin, S. E., et.al.,(2012). Health benefits of gastric bypass surgery after 6 years. *JAMA, 308*(11), 1122–1131. https://doi.org/10.1001/2012.jama.11164

37  Colquitt, J. L., Pickett, K., Loveman, E., & Frampton, G. K. (2014). Surgery for weight loss in adults. *The Cochrane database of systematic reviews, 2014*(8), CD003641. https://doi.org/10.1002/14651858.CD003641.pub4

38  Sjöström, L., Peltonen, M., Jacobson, P.,et.al., (2012). Bariatric surgery and long-term cardiovascular events. *JAMA, 307*(1), 56–65. https://doi.org/10.1001/jama.2011.1914

39  Adams, T. D., Gress, R. E., Smith, S. C.,et.al.,(2007). Long-term mortality after gastric bypass surgery. *The New England journal of medicine, 357*(8), 753–761. https://doi.org/10.1056/NEJMoa066603

40  Chang, J., & Wittert, G. (2009). Effects of bariatric surgery on morbidity and mortality in severe obesity. *International journal of evidence-based healthcare, 7*(1), 43–48. https://doi.org/10.1111/j.1744-1609.2009.00123.x

41  Czupryniak, L., Strzelczyk, J., Cypryk, K., et.al.,(2004). Gastric bypass surgery in severely obese type 1 diabetic patients. *Diabetes care, 27*(10), 2561–2562. https://doi.org/10.2337/diacare.27.10.2561

# CHAPTER 9
# Metabolic Syndrome

The simplest way to look at all these associations, between obesity, heart disease, type 2 diabetes, metabolic syndrome, cancer, and Alzheimer's (not to mention the other the conditions that also associate with obesity and diabetes, such as gout, asthma, and fatty liver disease), is that what makes us fat - the quality and quantity of carbohydrates we consume - also makes us sick.
**Gary Taubes**

## Definition of Metabolic syndrome (MeS)

Metabolic syndrome is a term coined by Reaven in his seminal paper in 1988[1] and further expounded by many articles thereafter. It is also called the metabolic syndrome X (different from cardiac syndrome X) or Insulin resistance syndrome.

The term refers to a cluster of risk factors contributing to insulin resistance and the CVD (**Figure 9.1**). Different organisations (WHO, IDF, ATP III) have different criteria for diagnosis of MeS. The IDF and ATP III criteria are similar, except for the cut-offs for the waist circumferences among males and females. There is no evidence to suggest any advantages of one criterion over another.

The International Diabetes Federation 2006 criteria for metabolic syndrome requires two or more of the following:

- Waist circumference for male, ≥94 cm and, for female, ≥80 cm—required!
- Insulin resistance (fasting BM ≥5.6 mmol/l) WHO (fasting BM 6.1, PPG 7.8)
- HDL cholesterol for male, <1 mmol/L and, for female, <1.3 or on drug treatment for high cholesterol
- Triglyceride of ≥2 mmol/L or on drug treatment

---

### *Metabolic Syndrome*

A cluster of risk factors for development of insulin resistance and increased cardiovascular events include:

- Increased waist circumference
- Insulin resistance
- Dyslipidaemia

---

## Epidemiology of Metabolic Syndrome

Metabolic Syndrome (MeS) itself is not a single entity to measure. However, its clusters of criteria or risk factors making up the syndrome are rising globally as discussed in preceding chapters of this book. Therefore, MeS is generally on the rise in the world, driven by sedentary lifestyles and westernised lifestyles.

## Pathological and Clinical Significances of the Diagnosis of Metabolic Syndrome

The MeS does not have any peculiar pathogenesis underpinning the underlying insulin resistance. Instead, its individual risk factors that make up the syndrome contribute in their roles to increase the risks of insulin resistance and cardiovascular diseases.

Currently, there are debates about the clinical significance of the syndromic diagnosis and management as compared to management of its individual risk factors. Khan et.al, have highlighted that the syndromic diagnosis does not confer any clinical significance compared to the management of the individual risk factors. [1] This is based on the pathogenesis of the individual risk factor, lack of standardisation of the diagnostic criteria of MeS among different professional organisations, and different studies using different criteria. Further, the syndrome does not include newer risk factors for the development of the cardiovascular risks such as microalbuminuria, anaemia, and newer antipsychotic medications.

Personal clinical experience of the author suggests patients are more motivated to treatment and lifestyle modifications when approached in a syndromic way, rather than by way of individualistic risk factor management. In fact, studies have shown that, although tracking of the individual component is helpful, [3] tracking of the cluster of the components is better. [4]

## Management of Metabolic Syndrome (MeS)

The essence of management of MeS relates back to the quote by Gary Taubes. Management of MeS starts with addressing the increasing caloric intake and overcoming sedentary lifestyle, followed by addressing the individual clusters of risk factors widely described in the other chapters of this book, in the author's opinion, a syndromic approach.

## Risk of Cardiovascular Diseases in Metabolic Syndrome (MeS)

Many papers, including systematic reviews, show that obesity increases the risk of CVD. A paper published in the *Circulation Journal*, titled 'Metabolic Syndrome as a Precursor of Cardiovascular Disease and Type 2 Diabetes Mellitus', where 3,323 middle-aged adults without CVD and diabetes were followed up over eight years, has shown that metabolic syndrome was associated with increased incidences of both CVD and diabetes. [5] The risk was higher among males compared to females.

## Childhood Metabolic Syndrome (MeS)

It is becoming increasingly common to see obese children everywhere, and it is no different in the developing world.

The IDF paper on childhood metabolic syndrome acknowledges that childhood metabolic syndrome is a rising public health concern worldwide. [6, 7] The co-author reiterates, 'This generation is going to die before their parents,' and implores governments throughout the world to make necessary environmental changes that will help address this rising trend.

Further, the document states that metabolic syndrome in childhood must be diagnosed among those within the age groups of 10 to 16 years of age. Those under 10 years old should not be diagnosed, and those above 16 years old should be classified as adult metabolic syndrome.

Those under 10 years old should be diagnosed with abdominal obesity using waist circumference percentiles and not absolute values. This is to compensate for childhood developmental and ethnicity variations.

**Diagnostic criteria for childhood (11 to 16 years old) metabolic syndrome by IDF, therefore, is:**

1. Abdominal obesity by waist circumference in percentiles plus ≥2 of the remaining variables
2. Elevated triglyceride
3. Low HDL
4. High BP
5. Prediabetes or Diabetes

## Key Messages:

- **MeS is a cluster of conditions that contribute to increasing cardiovascular diseases.**
- **A syndromic approach to management is shown to be helpful in reduction of cardiovascular diseases.**
- **Childhood MeS is rising and is diagnosed by the IDF diagnostic criteria.**

## References

1  Gerald M Reaven. Role of Insulin Resistance in Human Disease. Diabetes 1988 Dec; 37(12): 1595-1607.https://doi.org/10.2337/diab.37.12.1595

2  Kahn, R., Buse, J., Ferrannini, E., Stern, M., American Diabetes Association, & European Association for the Study of Diabetes (2005). The metabolic syndrome: time for a critical appraisal: joint statement from the American Diabetes Association and the European Association for the Study of Diabetes. *Diabetes care, 28*(9), 2289–2304. https://doi.org/10.2337/diacare.28.9.2289

3  Webber, L. S., Srinivasan, S. R., Wattigney, W. A., & Berenson, G. S. (1991). Tracking of serum lipids and lipoproteins from childhood to adulthood. The Bogalusa Heart Study. *American journal of epidemiology, 133*(9), 884–899. https://doi.org/10.1093/oxfordjournals.aje.a115968

4  Bao, W., Srinivasan, S. R., Wattigney, W. A., & Berenson, G. S. (1994). Persistence of multiple cardiovascular risk clustering related to syndrome X from childhood to young adulthood. The Bogalusa Heart Study. *Archives of internal medicine, 154*(16), 1842–1847.

5  Wilson, P. W., D'Agostino, R. B., Parise, H., Sullivan, L., & Meigs, J. B. (2005). Metabolic syndrome as a precursor of cardiovascular disease and type 2 diabetes mellitus. *Circulation, 112*(20), 3066–3072. https://doi.org/10.1161/CIRCULATIONAHA.105.539528

6  IDF definition of Childhood & Adolescent Metabolic Syndrome. http://www.idf.org/metabolic-syndrome/children

7  Zimmet, P., Alberti, K. G., Kaufman, F., Tajima, N., Silink, M., Arslanian, S., Wong, G., Bennett, P., Shaw, J., Caprio, S., & IDF Consensus Group (2007). The metabolic syndrome in children and adolescents - an IDF consensus report. *Pediatric diabetes, 8*(5), 299–306. https://doi.org/10.1111/j.1399-5448.2007.00271.x.

# CHAPTER 10

# Behaviour and Psychological Management of Diabetes Mellitus

We change other people's behaviour by changing our own!
**Anonymous**

## Behavioural Aspects of Diabetes Prevention

T2DM is a lifestyle disease marked by unconscious and persistent indulgence in lifestyle behaviours that ultimately lead to the development of the condition.

The aspects and stages of these behaviours are explained by different psychosocial models. It is assumed that understanding of these models will help a healthcare worker to be in a strong position to offer appropriate help to the patients, leading to the change of their destructive behaviours, which can control and even remit their diabetes.

These models can also be applied in other situations where people's behaviour poses risks to themselves, their communities and societies.

### Social Cognitive Theory (SCT)

SCT is one of the theories advanced by Albert Bandura to understand the process of behaviour among people. It suggests that people's behaviour is shaped by their environments (people and culture), cognition, and internal predisposition. [1]

This theory explains that a person learns the behaviour from observing other people's behaviour in the society they live. They become conditioned with repetition and cultured with acceptance by the society. For example, if a behaviour is tolerated and or accepted by any societies, it will be widely accepted and practiced, even though it may be unhealthy. Secondly personal dispositions among people can be deemed unhealthy, and this is not by choice but by ignorance.

Understanding the influence of the different factors (environment, culture, and individual predisposition) determining human behaviour can make it easy to address these factors. And that can lead to effecting change in their destructive behaviours for the better.

### Health Belief Model (HBM)

The HBM is another of the psychosocial models that proposes that, if people at risk of developing diabetes are made aware of their risky behaviours and the seriousness of those risks, there would be an inclination towards change to avert the perils of diabetes.

Historical Perspective of Health Belief Model (HBM)

In the 1950s, prevention of diseases somewhat took precedence over curative work. People were offered tests that were merely demonstrative in nature or done in small numbers or at low costs. There was an overarching tendency at that time for the public to ignore the preventative education. This led to research into the development of a theory to address patients' preventative healthy behaviour. Such a theory would have to involve dealing with the behaviour of people who were not suffering disabling disease and stressed the importance of consequences of behaviour in predicting patients' actions. [2, 3]

The HBM has several stages that allows understanding of patients' illness susceptibility and behaviours leading to adverse outcomes. These are:

1. Perceived susceptibility—patients' judgement of their risk of contracting the disease
2. Seriousness—patients' judgement of the seriousness of the illness arising from their behaviours
3. Solutions—patients' willingness to change their behaviours due to the risk posed by the seriousness of the disease
4. Perceived benefits—patients' belief in the efficacy of the advised action to reduce risk or seriousness of impact
5. Barriers—the barriers, as perceived by patients, to behavioural change
6. Cues to action—HCP strategising how to address patients' behavioural change
7. Self-efficacy—patients' confidence in their abilities to act

With this information, a health care practitioner (HCP) can offer options and support for patients in their decision-making process.

## Transtheoretical Model (Change Model)

This model is also called the change model and was developed by Prochaska and DiClemente in 1977 to determine the readiness of a person to intentionally change his or her behaviour. [4] It has six stages of change (**Figure 10.1**) and was used to determine why some smokers quit smoking intentionally whilst others needed support to change. [5] The six stages of change are

- Precontemplation
- Contemplation
- Preparation
- Action
- Maintenance
- Termination.

Precontemplation

In this stage, people lack information about the consequences and the seriousness of their behaviours to themselves and to others. They manifest avoidance, contempt, and ignorance. They are highly unlikely to change when in this stage.

Contemplation Stage

Individuals at this stage are intending to change and are aware of the positive and negative impacts of their behaviour and the need for change within the next six months. Counselling in this stage can reinforce patients' decision to change their destructive behaviour.

## Preparation

At this stage, individuals decide to act in the immediate future, which is usually a month. They have a plan of action, start to take a few steps towards changing behaviour and believe this will have a positive impact on their lives.

## Action

This is the stage when the individuals have made modifications in their lives in the last six months and intend to keep moving with that positive change.

## Maintenance

Individuals in this stage work to prevent relapses and put less emphasis on applying frequent change process at this stage.

## Termination

This is the final stage. At this point, individuals have no desire to go back to the unhealthy behaviour and are confident they will not relapse.

It is particularly important to bear these stages in mind when interacting with patients for whom behavioural change is needed. Knowing which stage they are stuck at enables a support person to better assist them in changing their behaviours. The processes of rolling, negotiation, and developing a shared plan of management are part of the motivational counselling techniques propounded by Rollnick et al.[6]

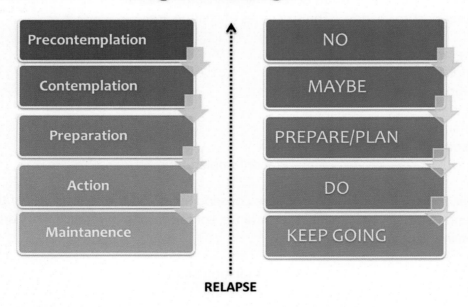

**Figure 10.1** The transtheoretical or change model: Stages of changes and possible outcome. Reproduced with permission from *Wikipedia*.

## Motivational Counselling

Motivational Counselling is a strategy developed by Rollnick to address patients' uncertainty about a particular behavioural change, increasing their awareness of the benefits of the change and providing motivation for them to embark on the behaviour change.[6] It is a way of directing patients to make lifestyle changes by providing guidance during the counselling process with regular follow-ups.

Unlike traditional counselling, where patients were lectured about their conditions and the need to change, this method takes a different approach—enabling the patient to be the focus in the decision-making process.

A systematic analysis has shown that those who receive motivational counselling are better at changing their lifestyles compared with those who do not.[7] It is an effective, evidence-based, and patient-centred approach to counselling patients on behaviour changes and comprises of four key elements—expressing empathy, rolling with resistance, developing discrepancy, and supporting self-efficacy.

### Express empathy through active listening

Physicians can ask for permission prior to offering advice a patient has not asked for, which shows respect and empowers the patient.

### Roll with resistance

Avoid argument and try to understand patients' unwillingness to change.

### Develop discrepancy

Patients' misunderstanding or incorrect beliefs needed to be corrected.

### Support self-efficacy:

Patients need to have the confidence that they can achieve success at making change. Empowering people and providing options are keys for self-efficacy. Patients come up with solutions themselves, instead of their doctor prescribing solutions to them.

---

**Psychosocial models are used to:**

- **Understand and explain the reasons people engage in destructive lifestyle behaviours that lead to diabetes (social cognitive theory)**
- **Attempt to categorise the stages of changes of these behaviours (transtheoretical change model)**
- **Discover ideas about and understanding of the risky behaviours of patients, support them to identify their barriers to change, and allow them to find their own solutions (health belief model)**
- **Listen, roll, and develop discrepancy and facilitate self-efficacy, which allows those who are uncertain to be certain about their change of behaviour (motivational counselling)**

# Psychological Issues in Diabetes Patients

Like all chronic and progressive diseases, diabetes has social, psychological, and emotional aspects that require address by the patient and his or her health carer. These psychological issues can be so enormous and devastating to patients that they are unable to care for themselves, resulting in worsening of their diabetes and its complications.

The DAWN (Diabetes Attitudes, Wishes, and Needs) studies in the early 2000s were an attempt to identify the attitudes, wishes, and needs of the diabetic patients. [8, 9]

DAWN 1 showed that adherence to treatment prescription among diabetes patients (both T1DM & T2DM) were low. And patients had high psychosocial stress levels related to the diagnosis, with only 3.3% of the patients receiving some form of psychological care and support. [8]

DAWN 2 attempted to identify psychosocial outcomes of diabetic patients globally. It showed that 85.2% of all newly diagnosed diabetes patients have negative grieving reactions of shock, guilt, anger, anxiety, depression, and helplessness related to the diagnosis. The rates of depression and other psychological difficulties are higher among people with diabetes and obese people seeking treatment compared to those without diabetes. [9]. Depression affects 20 to 25% of patients with diabetes and is also associated with an increased risk of myocardial infarction and all-cause mortality. [10] Addressing these psychological issues are key in alleviating the effect of mood or anxiety disorders on the performance of health-maintenance routines, improvement in control of brittle diabetes, improving quality of life and reducing myocardial infarction. [11]

## Management of Psychological Issues

### Early Management at The Time of Diagnosis

Recognising the grieving reactions at the time of diagnosis is particularly important for the health provider, who can be able to assist patients in overcoming these stages quickly and to enhance concentration on their chronic self-management of diabetes. Support at this period can vary, but essentially, the HCP will have to:

- Reassure patients that it's normal to react to the bad news and that diabetes, although it's a chronic progressive disease, is manageable, and patients can be able to enjoy quality of life
- Provide emotional support at the time of grief
- Answer all questions and doubts raised by the patients
- Offer to refer patients to appropriate counsellors and diabetic educators and nurses should they need further support
- Offer to provide review and further psychological and emotional support during reviews and consultations as appropriate

The specific grief reactions can be handled in these suggested ways:

- Denial can be addressed with positive regard and professional tone that conveys sincere acceptance in spite of shortcomings.

- Anger and shame can be addressed by letting patients know it was not their fault, nor the faults of others that they have diabetes and that treatments are effective to control and prevent the short and the longterm complications.
- Grief can be addressed by acknowledging that grief is normal but must be overcome quickly to focus on the long-term challenges. Patients can invoke inner strength to face the challenge when motivated and supported wholesomely.

Furthermore, the HCP can describe the condition and the pathophysiology, risk factors, complications and short and long-term management plan. Assess patient using HBM and provide support and guidance as to what the patient can do and advise that future insulin is not a treatment failure but a control mechanism that will inevitably happen. Allow and create an environment where patients feel comfortable in expressing their ideas, fears, and concerns.

### Kübler - Ross Model of Grief Reactions

- Denial
- Anger
- Bargaining
- Depression
- Acceptance

Continuous Management of Psychological Issues After Diagnosis

The initial reactions to the diagnosis of diabetes can vary among patients according to the Kübler - Ross stages of grief reactions—denial, anger, bargaining, depression, and acceptance.

Patients' degree of reactions can vary widely. Some take their diagnosis very lightly, while others may be severely affected.

Psychosocial assessment can be routinely done at time of diagnosis; during regular visits; during hospitalisation; at onset of a new complication; and when the patient is having issues with glycaemic control, quality of life, or self-management. Patients are considered more susceptible to psychological problems at diagnosis when they develop a new complication or when treatment needs to be intensified. [12]

Ongoing Long-Term Psychological Management

ADA recommends routine screening for psychosocial problems that include depression, anxiety, and diabetes-related distress as part of the ongoing management of diabetes. [13] Older individuals, 65 years old and up, with diabetes are considered high priority for depression screening and treatment.

The Depression Anxiety Stress Scales (DASS) is a forty-two-point screening test that can be used to screen for depression and anxiety in clinics. [14]

## Key Messages:

- **Unhealthy behaviours leading to diabetes can be addressed through several social behavioural models.**
- **Individuals who are uncertain about their own risky behaviours can be supported through the process of motivational counselling.**
- **It's important to understand the grief reactions of the newly diagnosed diabetes and be prepared to support patients through the process to reduce long term complications.**

## References:

1   Bandura A. (2004). Health promotion by social cognitive means. *Health education & behavior: the official publication of the Society for Public Health Education, 31*(2), 143–164. https://doi.org/10.1177/1090198104263660.

2   Jones and Bartlett Learning. Health Belief Model. https://www.jblearning.com..

3   *Health Belief Model. https://www.utwente.nl*

4   Behavioural Change Models. The Transtheoretical Model (Stages of Changes) Boston University School of Public Health. (2013). https://www.sphweb.bumc.bu.edu/otlt/MPH-Modules/SB/SB721-Models/SB721-Models6.html.

5   Velicer, W. F., Prochaska, J. O., Fava, J. L., Norman, G. J., & Redding, C. A. (1998). Smoking cessation and stress management: Applications of the transtheoretical model of behavior change. Homeostasis in Health and Disease, 38, 216-233.

6   S Rollnick, WR Miller and CC Butler. Motivational Interviewing in Health Care: Helping Patients Change Behavior. New York, New York: The Guilford Press. 2008. 210. ISBN-13:978-1-59.85-612-0.

7   Frost, H., Campbell, P., Maxwell, M., O'Carroll, R. E., Dombrowski, S. U., Williams, B., Cheyne, H., Coles, E., & Pollock, A. (2018). Effectiveness of Motivational Interviewing on adult behaviour change in health and social care settings: A systematic review of reviews. *PloS one, 13*(10), e0204890. https://doi.org/10.1371/journal.pone.0204890

8   Skovlund, S. E., & Peyrot, M. (2005). The Diabetes Attitudes, Wishes, and Needs (DAWN) program: A new approach to improving outcomes of diabetes care. *Diabetes Spectrum, 18*(3), 136-142. https://doi.org/10.2337/diaspect.18.3.136

9   Nicolucci, A., Kovacs Burns, K., Holt, R. I.,et.al., & DAWN2 Study Group (2013). Diabetes Attitudes, Wishes and Needs second study (DAWN2™): cross-national benchmarking of diabetes-related psychosocial outcomes for people with diabetes. *Diabetic medicine: a journal of the British Diabetic Association, 30*(7), 767–777. https://doi.org/10.1111/dme.12245.

10  Scherrer, J. F., Garfield, L. D., Chrusciel, T., et.al.,(2011). Increased risk of myocardial infarction in depressed patients with type 2 diabetes. *Diabetes care, 34*(8), 1729–1734. https://doi.org/10.2337/dc11-0031

11  Gavard, J. A., Lustman, P. J., & Clouse, R. E. (1993). Prevalence of depression in adults with diabetes. An epidemiological evaluation. *Diabetes care, 16*(8), 1167–1178. https://doi.org/10.2337/diacare.16.8.

12  Fisher, L., Hessler, D. M., Polonsky, W. H., & Mullan, J. (2012). When is diabetes distress clinically meaningful? establishing cut points for the Diabetes Distress Scale. *Diabetes care, 35*(2), 259–264. https://doi.org/10.2337/dc11-1572

13  American Diabetes Association (2022). Introduction: Standards of Medical Care in Diabetes-2022. *Diabetes care, 45*(Suppl 1), S1–S2. https://doi.org/10.2337/dc22-Sint

14  Health Focus. Depression Anxiety and Stress Scale DASS (-42). https://www.healthfocuspsychology.com.au/tools/dass-42.

# CHAPTER 11
# Healthcare Models in Clinical Practice

*The outcomes we are getting from our healthcare are dictated by
economic incentives put in place a long time ago.*
**Unknown**

## Acute Care Clinical Model

The acute care clinical model is a form of care model that integrates all cadres of services within a healthcare system, where the provision of acute care is followed by the termination of the services relationship with the patient after the care.

Such services include screening in a single point in time and assessment of the condition leading to possible admission with a short course of minimal treatment or brief care. This is followed by discharge and the termination of the service relationship.

This clinical care model is offered in the emergencies department and in acute and other specialty wards of secondary care settings. Diabetic patients receive care in this model during their diagnosis and management of their acute complications. Most of their care is otherwise undertaken under the chronic clinical care model.

## Chronic Care Model (CCM)

Chronic medical conditions are defined in different ways, but a simple definition would be 'conditions that require ongoing or lifelong treatments.[1] These conditions are managed under the chronic care model, which encompasses the patient's safety and information, community resourcing and support, healthcare delivery system, and the care coordination between these systems.

A Cochrane review by Renders et al. in 2001 concluded that a combination of multiple strategies is the most effective way of improving chronic disease care, and the chronic care model is an example of such care.[2]

### Historical Perspective of the CCM

The CCM was developed at the MacColl Center for Health Care Innovation in Washington, USA; reviewed in 1997; and tested in 1998 across different healthcare settings, which led to the creation of Improving Chronic Illness Care Program.

Refinements of the CCM was carried out by Improving Chronic Illness Care team in 2003, which included the following initial themes:

- Patient safety (in Health System)
- Cultural competency (in Delivery System Design)
- Care coordination (in Health System and Clinical Information Systems)
- Community policies (in Community Resources and Policies) and
- Case management (in Delivery System Design).

## Application of CCM

The CCM has been trialled in many chronic illnesses and has been shown to improve patient outcomes. Several trials in diabetes management in both the developing and the developed world have shown consistencies in improved patient outcomes. A study in the Philippines using the pre-existing health systems services has shown CCM to improve the clinical endpoints.[3] A systematic review of CCM integrated in the primary care settings in the United States has also shown positive outcomes.[4]

The CCM involves not only the patient and the healthcare provider but also the society/community in which the patient lives and the healthcare system to improve the outcome. This is a holistic approach that involves a societal and healthcare system context.

## Requirements for Optimal Chronic Care Model

Several factors contribute to a reliable and effective delivery of the chronic care model in the communities for patients who have chronic illnesses. These factors are:

- Community policies and resources—local community health facilities must have provisions and staff to care for patients with chronic medical conditions such as diabetes
- Health care organisation—presence of health care close to the communities with adequate qualified staff and resources improves outcomes
- Clinical information systems—having an interconnected information system ensures patient medical information is easily accessible for improved care
- Decision support and delivery system—providing evidenced-based advice, decisions, and involving patients in their own care

# Patient Empowerment

> The 'doctor is the expert on the condition ... but the patient is an expert on himself ...' i.e., the patient knows their life, the barriers they face, the ways to overcome these perceived barriers and the willingness to do it. Our job as doctors and HCPs is to try and find a way to help them facilitate this: in a 'patient-centred approach'.
> **Unknown**

Patient Empowerment is, therefore, the process in which the HCP empowers patients with chronic diseases such as diabetes to be knowledgeable and self-confident and to able to make informed decisions on the care of their chronic conditions. It encompasses the 'patient-centred care', where patients are deemed the centre of all decisions by the healthcare professionals. In fact, ADA and EASD 2012 Position Statement recommends a patient-centred approach to management of diabetes.[5] The process involves the healthcare worker providing:

- All important and necessary information through education
- Guidance on the decision related to management of the diseases
- Support for the patients in their decisions, regardless of the choices they make

This process requires both patients and doctors to adopt new roles. The patient is seen as the 'sage on the stage', whilst the health professional is a 'guide on the side-line'.

## Benefits of Patient Empowerment

Patient empowerment benefits both patients and their healthcare providers and, therefore, is very important for both parties to spare some time towards this process. The benefits are many.

### Patients' Benefits

- A greater understanding of the illness
- The ability to better communicate with their HCP
- Greater satisfaction with healthcare
- Improved metabolic, psychosocial, and emotional well-being

### Healthcare Providers' (HCP's) Benefits

- Achievement of recommended standards or targets of care
- Improved outcomes
- Personal and professional satisfaction
- Increased motivation in care of patients

## Time or No Time for Patient Empowerment

Newly diagnosed diabetic patients react differently to the bad news. Reactions may include denial, anger, bargaining, and depression and, finally, acceptance. Counselling is particularly an important tool to help patients overcome these emotional stages of reactions and empower them to manage their diabetes . The DAWN study found 85% of patients suffer shock, guilt, anger, anxiety, depression, and helplessness related to a diagnosis of diabetes. Moreover the patients' initial poor reaction to the diagnosis of diabetes led to poorer outcomes in terms of glycaemic control than those with good reactions. [6]

Woodcock et al., however, noted that patient-centred care improved both glycemic and psychological outcomes. [7] Further, Polonsky et al. found that patients who had good experiences at the time of their diagnoses, along with clear action plans to manage their conditions, suffered less distress and had better diabetes management in the first five years post diagnosis. [8]

It is, however, interesting to note that the nurses trained in patient-centred care in the Woodcock study found that there was not enough time to deliver the intervention well, and their confidence in delivering the intervention decreased throughout the trial period. The challenge now is to overcome this issue at all levels of healthcare so that diabetic patients will be empowered to start an enjoyable journey of long-term self-care.

---

**This philosophy of patient empowerment essentially involves well-informed patients working as partners with a knowledgeable qualified team who possess expertise, equipment, and resources to deliver and provide guidance in the self-management of diabetic patients. The empowerment philosophy creates partnership and truly facilitates patient-centred care.**

---

# Diabetes Self-Education Management (DSEM)

"Little knowledge is a dangerous thing; the Diabetic who knows the most lives the longest"
**Elliot P. Joslin, 1929**

### Structured Diabetes Education Programme

Education of diabetes patient forms the fundamental basis for patient empowerment. Diabetes education is evidenced based and has been shown to:

- Improve glycaemic control—reduces HBA1c by 1% at six months to 0.5% at one year
- Improve QoL
- Improve treatment satisfaction
- Reduce smoking cessation
- Reduce depression and weight
- Improve understanding of diabetes
- Reduces hypoglycaemia

Education must be structured. The National Institute of Clinical Excellence (NICE) criteria for a structured education are:[9]

- Written curriculum
- Delivered by trained educators
- Quality assured
- Audited

The aims of education programmes in diabetes are essentially to:

- Minimise chronic complications
- Reduce risk factors for diabetes
- Benefit patients' quality of life

There are three types of self-education programmes for diabetes patients to aid in their self-management:

1. DAFNE education programme
2. DESMOND education programme
3. X-PERT education programme

Dose Adjustment for Normal Eating (DAFNE)

DAFNE stands for **D**ose **A**djustment **f**or **N**ormal **E**ating and is an education programme for management of T1DM in adults, where they are taught the skills necessary to estimate the carbohydrate in each meal and to inject the right dose of insulin.

DAFNE was first introduced in Germany in 1970 and was adopted by the United Kingdom. Several studies have shown that DAFNE had better outcomes than other education approaches among the T1DM patients and therefore, this education strategy has been adopted globally.

The programme involves attending a full five-day training course, plus a follow-up session around eight weeks after the course. The structured teaching programme is delivered to groups of six to eight participants under the supervision of DAFNE-trained educators, where insulin dosage is adjusted according to the amount of carbohydrate eaten. The insulin sensitivity factor, often called the insulin correction factor is used in the advanced carbohydrate counting. This is where 1 unit of insulin is estimated to drop glucose in a fasting or premeal state over two to four hours.

Correction factor = 100/TDD
TDD = total daily dose (basal + boluses)

A study has shown that DAFNE has improved patients' confidence in adjusting their insulin doses and motivation in their own care. However, the long-term follow-up showed that only a minority had maintained their confidences in adjusting their insulin dosages. Many felt the need to be reviewed by their HCP and endorsement of their decisions. [10] However, a randomised control trial involving 169 patients in an English secondary care diabetic clinics showed improved quality of life and glycaemic control in people with type 1 diabetes without worsening severe hypoglycaemia or cardiovascular risk. [11]

## Diabetes Education and Self-Management for Newly Diagnosed Diabetes (DESMOND)

DESMOND is the self-management education programme for those patients with T2DM. It stands for **D**iabetes **E**ducation and **S**elf-**M**anagement for **N**ewly **D**iagnosed **D**iabetes.

It is a set of education programmes that enables participants to be educated to increase their understanding about diabetes and glycaemic controls, share self-management skills, and come out empowered with sets of goals to achieve diabetes control and improve their overall health and well-being.

A randomised controlled trial in the United Kingdom, published in *The BMJ* showed that DESMOND, for patients with newly diagnosed type 2 diabetes, resulted in greater improvements in weight loss, smoking cessation and positive improvements in beliefs about illness compared with those who did not participate in DESMOND. However, there was no difference in haemoglobin A1c levels up to twelve months after diagnosis [12]

## X-PERT Programme

The X-PERT structured education programme is delivered over six weeks by HCPs who have trained in this program as educators. The programme is designed to increase participants' knowledge, skills, and confidence to make informed decisions and self-manage their condition.

The X-PERT programme includes X-PERT Diabetes, X-PERT Insulin and X-POD. These structured education programmes deliver a range of topics to help people understand:

- Health and disease
- Tablets and insulin
- Food, nutrients, and digestion
- What health results mean
- The benefit of physical activity
- Weight management
- The impact of blood glucose, blood pressure, and blood cholesterol levels on long-term health
- Self-management of diabetes
- Special considerations regarding travel

The X-PERT programmes have been shown in a randomised controlled trial to improve clinical, lifestyle, and psychosocial outcomes in white Caucasian and South Asian people with newly diagnosed and existing diabetes. [13] They have also been demonstrated to be a cost-effective strategy in the treatment and management of diabetes; it costs as little as £15 per participant and has the potential to reduce the NHS prescription bill by £367 million per year. [14]

---

**Three Types of Diabetes Education Programmes**

1. **DAFNE—carbohydrate estimation education programme in T1DM for insulin dose adjustment**
2. **DESMOND—a programme designed to increase patients' knowledge, self-management skills, and empowerment to achieve glycaemic control with improved well being**
3. **X-PERT—comprehensive sets of education and training programmes for patients with both types of diabetes**

---

## Key Messages:

- **Diabetes is a chronic progressive disease that requires care in a chronic care model. Its acute complications are managed under the acute care model.**
- **Patient empowerment through education allows patients to manage their diabetes safely, improves outcomes and reduces costs to patients and healthcare systems alike.**

## References:

1   Improving Chronic Illnesses. The Chronic Care Module. https://www.improvingchroniccare.org/index.php?p...Chronic_CareModel&s...
2   Renders, C. M., Valk, G. D., Griffin, S. J., Wagner, E. H., Eijk Van, J. T., & Assendelft, W. J. (2001). Interventions to improve the management of diabetes in primary care, outpatient, and community settings: a systematic review. *Diabetes care*, *24*(10), 1821–1833. https://doi.org/10.2337/diacare.24.10.
3   Ku, G. M., & Kegels, G. (2014). Integrating chronic care with primary care activities: enriching healthcare staff knowledge and skills and improving glycemic control of a cohort of people with diabetes through the First Line Diabetes Care Project in the Philippines. *Global health action*, 7, 25286. https://doi.org/10.3402/gha.v7.25286.
4   Stellefson, M., Dipnarine, K., & Stopka, C. (2013). The chronic care model and diabetes management in US primary care settings: a systematic review. *Preventing chronic disease*, *10*, E26. https://doi.org/10.5888/pcd10.
5   Inzucchi, S. E., Bergenstal, R. M., Buse, J. B.,et.al., American Diabetes Association (ADA), & European Association for the Study of Diabetes (EASD) (2012). Management of hyperglycemia in type 2 diabetes: a patient-centered approach: position statement of the American Diabetes Association (ADA) and the European Association for the Study of Diabetes (EASD). *Diabetes care*, *35*(6), 1364–1379. https://doi.org/10.2337/dc12-0413.
6   Soren E. Skovlund, Mark Peyrot, on behalf of the DAWN International Advisory Panel; The Diabetes Attitudes, Wishes, and Needs (DAWN) Program: A New Approach to Improving Outcomes of Diabetes Care. *Diabetes Spectr* 1 July 2005; 18 (3): 136–142. https://doi.org/10.2337/diaspect.18.3.136
7   Woodcock, A. J., Kinmonth, A. L., Campbell, M. J., Griffin, S. J., & Spiegal, N. M. (1999). Diabetes care from diagnosis: effects of training in patient-centred care on beliefs, attitudes and behaviour of primary care professionals. *Patient education and counseling*, *37*(1), 65–79. https://doi.org/10.1016/s0738-3991(98)00104-9.
8   Polonsky, W. H., Fisher, L., Guzman, S., Sieber, W. J., Philis-Tsimikas, A., & Edelman, S. V. (2010). Are patients' initial experiences at the diagnosis of type 2 diabetes associated with attitudes and self-management over time?. *The Diabetes educator*, *36*(5), 828–834. https://doi.org/10.1177/0145721710378539

9    Patient Education Models: Guidance', NICE (2003). https://www.publications.nice.org.uk/type-2-diabetes-cg87/guidance#patient-education,

10   Lawton, J., Rankin, D., Cooke, D., Elliott, J., Amiel, S., Heller, S., & UK NIHR DAFNE Study Group (2012). Patients' experiences of adjusting insulin doses when implementing flexible intensive insulin therapy: a longitudinal, qualitative investigation. *Diabetes research and clinical practice, 98*(2), 236–242. https://doi.org/10.1016/j.diabres.2012.09.024

11   DAFNE Study Group (2002). Training in flexible, intensive insulin management to enable dietary freedom in people with type 1 diabetes: dose adjustment for normal eating (DAFNE) randomised controlled trial. *BMJ (Clinical research ed.), 325*(7367), 746. https://doi.org/10.1136/bmj.325.7367.746

12   Davies, M. J., Heller, S., Skinner, T. C.,et.al., & Diabetes Education and Self Management for Ongoing and Newly Diagnosed Collaborative (2008). Effectiveness of the diabetes education and self management for ongoing and newly diagnosed (DESMOND) programme for people with newly diagnosed type 2 diabetes: cluster randomised controlled trial. *BMJ (Clinical research ed.), 336*(7642), 491–495. https://doi.org/10.1136/bmj.39474.922025.BE

13   Deakin, T. A., Cade, J. E., Williams, R., & Greenwood, D. C. (2006). Structured patient education: the diabetes X-PERT Programme makes a difference. *Diabetic medicine : a journal of the British Diabetic Association, 23*(9), 944–954. https://doi.org/10.1111/j.1464-

14   T. A. Deakin, 'The Diabetes Pandemic: Is Structured Education the Solution or an Unnecessary Expense?' *Pract Diabetes*, 28 (2011a), 358–61.

# CHAPTER 12

# Living with Diabetes

Life is not about waiting for the storm to pass. It's about how to dance in the rain.
**Vivien Greene**

## Diabetes in Pregnancy

The prevalence of diabetes in pregnancy has been increasing worldwide commensurate with the increasing diabetes epidemic.

Pre-pregnancy screening and treating this group of pregnant women through counselling and strict lifestyle modifications with good glycaemic control before pregnancy has been shown to reduce maternal and neonatal complications such as pre-eclampsia, macrosomia, caesarean section, foetal shoulder dystocia, and foetal death. Further, hypertension, obesity, and diabetes among off springs are reduced.[1] Postpartum follow-up and management of patients can lead to better outcomes.

### Pathophysiology

Pregnancy generally is a diabetogenic condition that can worsen glycaemic control among those who have pre-gestation diabetes or increase risks of overt hyperglycaemia among high-risk women.

Pregnancy, in simplistic terms, has an early anabolic stage of building up energy reserves (increased fat and energy storages) for fetoplacental and maternal needs in the last trimester. Insulin secretion increases during the first trimester with a drop in its resistance, however, its sensitivity remains the same. This is the period where hypoglycaemia can occur if patients are treated with insulin. Close monitoring will prevent this.

The catabolic state starts in the second and third trimesters of the pregnancy. The placental steroids and proteins tend to antagonise the insulin effects and, therefore, increase insulin resistance. There are additional insulin-antagonising effects of increased adipokine secretions leading to lipolysis and increased hyperglycaemia. The need for exogenous insulin increases here because hyperglycaemia ensures and can cause maternal and foetal complications.

Regular reviews of pregnant women with diabetes are important to optimally assess the changing insulin sensitivity and manage glycaemic fluctuations.

---

### Insulin Sensitivity and Resistances during the Stages of Pregnancy

- First trimester (anabolic state)
  Insulin sensitivity remains the same, but its resistance drops increasing risk of hypoglycaemia

- Second and third trimesters (catabolic state)
  Insulin drops and its resistance increases, increasing risk of hyperglycaemia

**Insulin Management of Overt Diabetes in Pregnancy**

The American College of Obstetrics and Gynaecology (ACOG) has released a position paper on the management of this group of pregnant women, which is summarised below. [2]

### Dietary Management

The ACOG advises carbohydrate counting and bedtime snacks for women to prevent nocturnal hypoglycaemia. Females are advised to reduce calories (those with normal weight to 30 to 35 kCal/kg/day and those with weight of >120kg to 24 kCal/kg/day) to maintain a sugar level of four to six. In the opinion of the author, this sugar range is too tight and quiet often difficult to attain. Therefore, at least a sugar level of five to eight is acceptable.

### Preconception

Optimal glycaemic control for three months before conception is imperative in preventing pregnancy complications that could affect both the patient and her foetus. Counselling, lifestyle modifications, and optimal insulinisation are important part for achieving optimal glycaemic control.

Baseline investigations include microalbuminuria, fundoscopy, and ECG. Blood pressure must be checked, any abnormalities must be noted, and medical management must be optimised before pregnancy. Pregnancy can be advised at HBA1c level of <6.1 %. Patients with poorly controlled diabetes with HBA1c ≥9% must be discouraged to conceive until control is attained.

### Gestation

Insulin regimens are customised to achieve control. Optimal glycaemic control should be maintained, and frequent follow-up should be ensured to manage changing insulin needs. Insulin pump should be considered for select cases when glycaemic targets are difficult to achieve.

### Labour and Delivery

At the day of delivery, the morning insulin dose must be withheld; patient should be started on insulin infusion to maintain a blood glucose of 6 mmol/L. Normal insulin must be started at 1.25 units/hr, and if blood glucose drops below 4 mmol/L, then a dextrose infusion must be commenced.

### Postpartum

Reduce insulin to 50% of pre-delivery after satisfactory oral intake is achieved. Adjust insulin to attain optimal control and reduce the risk of hypoglycaemia, especially in patients who are breastfeeding.

## Gestational Diabetes Mellitus

Gestational diabetes is a term used to describe a transient state of hyperglycaemia that occurs during pregnancy among certain high-risk groups of patients. It can sometime predate pregnancy and often remits after delivery. However, having gestational diabetes increases the risks of development of overt diabetes later in life.

### Risk Factors of Developing Gestational Diabetes

- BMI > 30 kg/m$^2$
- Previous macrosomic baby weighing 4.5 kg or above
- Previous gestational diabetes
- First-degree relative with diabetes
- Family origin with high prevalence of diabetes (South Asian, black Caribbean, and Middle Eastern) as per NICE guidelines

### Management of High-Risk Patients for Diabetes (Prediabetes and GDM)

Identify these patients with high risk factors for developing gestational diabetes or diabetes, diagnose them, and initiate treatment using aggressive lifestyle modifications and pharmacotherapy to optimise glycaemic control before pregnancy to reduce complications for the mother and her foetus.

- Identify the risk factors for GDM

- Diagnosis of GDM:
  - High risk patients undergo screening with either a one-step or two-step OGTT at twelve weeks of gestation. Repeat the screen at twenty-four to twenty-six weeks if the first screen is negative.
  - Known GDM first screen at twenty-four to twenty-six weeks of gestation.

- Treat the Gestational Diabetes
  When to start treatment of GDM is often controversial. Studies show that treatment (lifestyle modifications, watchful control of glucose and insulin if deemed necessary) has reduced maternal and foetal complications such as pre-eclampsia, caesarean section, and macrosomia with shoulder dystocia respectively. [3, 4]

  Treatment can start with lifestyle modifications alone and monitoring of blood glucose. Personalised decisions must be made in starting treatment, which can include oral diabetic agents such as metformin and glyburide. Although these drugs are not approved for GDM and are known to cross the placenta, they have not been shown to affect the foetus in the short term. [5, 6] Patients can be counselled and informed of the lack of long-term effects before prescription.

  Insulin does not cross the placenta and is safe. Any available long or intermediate insulins can be prescribed as would be in a normal patient. Monitoring over the pregnancy should be done and adjustments made during periods of variability.

## Drinking Alcohol in Diabetes

### Alcohol in Diabetes Prevention

Alcohol in moderation protects patients from developing T2DM. A meta-analysis of thirteen studies by Carlsson et.al showed that moderate alcohol consumption has a protective effect from developing diabetes by 30%. [7] The 2010 Dietary Guidelines for Americans defines moderate alcohol consumption as the average daily consumption of up to one drink per day for women and up to two drinks per day for men and no more than three drinks in any single day for women and no more than four drinks in any single day for men. There were no protective effects from high alcohol consumption. Alcohol, however, is not a recommended therapy for prevention of diabetes.

*Effects of Alcohol in Diabetes*

Alcohol has several effects on metabolism. Some are related directly to the alcohol or its by-products (acetaldehyde or acetate), and others are due to the increase in NADH: NAD ratio.

NADH: NAD ratio inhibits gluconeogenesis. After consumption of 48 grams of alcohol, hepatic gluconeogenesis decreases by 48%, and glycogenolysis is impaired after alcohol consumption by 12%. These effects contribute to the hypoglycaemia that happens after hours of alcohol consumption. Furthermore, combination of carbohydrate and insulin can lead to reactive hypoglycaemia.[8]

*Advice to Patients with Diabetes*

As HCP, you can only advise diabetic patient on the risks of drinking alcohol but can't stop them from drinking socially. Patients can be told about the hypoglycaemic effects after hours of drinking to reduce basal insulin (analogues or NPH) and increase carbohydrate before drinking.

Further, patients who are self-monitoring BG should be warned of injecting prandial insulin in the transient hyperglycaemic state of drinking. Surely, the recommended levels are part of the information that should be delivered.

*Recommendation of Alcohol*

The NICE guideline recommends that men should not regularly drink more than three to four units of alcohol per day (maximum weekly intake of twenty-one units), and women no more than two to three units per day (maximum weekly intake of fourteen units).[9] Any amount more than that is excessive and can have short- and long-term consequences.

Thus, the emphasis is on encouraging moderate and sensible alcohol use in persons with diabetes if it is their choice to consume alcohol. If individuals with diabetes choose to consume alcohol, it should be in moderation and only by adults.

---

**Alcohol has a U-shaped relationship with diabetes, and this means:**

- **High alcohol acutely increases risk of hypoglycaemic complication**
- **Moderate alcohol prevents diabetes and even controls glycaemia**
- **Long-term excessive alcohol has more side effects**

**NICE and ADA recommendations is the same except in units of measurement:**

- **NICE quantifies minimum of fourteen units per week in females and twenty-one units per week for males.**
- **ADA says three bottles in a week for females and four per week for males.**

---

# Exercise with Diabetes

Evidence show that exercise improves glycaemic control, comorbid cardiovascular risk factors, and patients' quality of life. More diabetic patients today are living normal active lives as either amateurs or professionals in sports today than ever before. Although, exercise prescription is now an established management strategy among the diabetes, less is known of exercise prescription among the athletic population. [10] Recent observational studies and recommendations by professional organisations such as the ADA, NICE, and the National Athletic Trainers' Association (NATA) provide insight into ways to appropriately manage T1DM in athletic patients. In fact, this is a rising diabetic population, and providing appropriate levels of advice and care in this group is critically important before embarking on trainings.

All diabetic patients who wish to engage in moderate- to high-intensity exercises are advised to have a premedical check and assessment prior to engagement with specific advice to the patients and/or their trainers. This is to prevent complications that may arise from incorrect exercise regimen or fluctuations in blood glucose control.

Effective management plans require taking the following into consideration as recommended by Hornsby; [10]

- Demands of training and competition
- Athlete's goals
- Factors related to sports participation that may affect glucose homeostasis
- Safety of athletes' participation
- Adequate monitoring of blood glucose
- Types of exercises

## Demands of Training and Competition

Exercise essentially increases temperature and increases insulin sensitivity that could portend hypoglycaemia. Patients need to have a treatment strategy underpinned by insulin reduction before engaging in exercises. Pre-exercise, exercise and post-exercise glucose checks must be carried out to avoid post hypoglycaemic episodes.

Those with hyperglycaemia above 13 mmol/L should be advised not to engage in exercises until plasma glucose is within target levels prior to engagement. Engagement of HCP in understanding the types of exercises involved can allow optimal adjustments to treatment plans.

Athlete's Goals

Patients have different goals. Whatever the goals, appropriate and optimal management does not deviate from the norm. However, with competitive edge for enhanced performances, athletes can engage in scrupulous practices that can affect their glycaemic control. This means health workers need to be mindful of this issue when managing highly competitive athletes with huge sums of money in sight.

Factors Affecting Glucose Homeostasis

Pre-exercise blood sugar levels, intensity of exercise, and ambient environmental temperature all affect glucose homeostasis during exercises in both athletic and non-athletic T1DM patients engaging in any forms of exercises.

Safety of Athletes' Participation

All diabetes patients, including professional athletes, willing to engage in any forms of exercise prescription require a premedical assessment as advised by the ACSM and ACC to assess disabilities incurred by diabetes complications or other comorbidities before prescribing a particular individualised exercise prescription according to the values and needs of the patients. [11]

Pre-exercise, exercise, and post exercise glucose checks are fundamental parts of the safety measures taken in patient management. Staff involved in exercises should be taught the basics of diabetes and how to address complications arising from exercises.

Reviews of treatments are required regularly to optimise and stabilise patients for the long term.

## Types of Exercises

Aerobic exercises increase insulin sensitivity and reduce glucagon and other insulin-antagonising hormones. This increases the glucose consumption through increased uptake by the skeletal muscles, reduces glycogenolysis from the liver, and can lead to post exercise hypoglycaemia.

The risk of hypoglycaemia in moderate aerobic exercise is low since blood glucose is maintained by hepatic glycogenolysis. However, patients taking concomitant insulin and insulin secretagogues have potential risk of hypoglycaemia, and therefore, insulin reduction should be considered.

Anaerobic exercises on the other hand, increase catecholamines but reduces insulin sensitivity. This causes a reduction in the glucose uptake by the skeletal muscle and increases glucose production through glycogenolysis. This can lead to post exercise hyperglycaemia (**Figure 12.1**).

| Type of Exercise | Description | Effects on Glucose |
|---|---|---|
| **Aerobic** | **Longer duration**<br>**Lower intensity**<br>**e.g., Running, cycling** | **Drops glucose levels** |
| **Anaerobic** | **Shorter duration**<br>**Higher intensity**<br>**e.g., Weightlifting** | **Spikes glucose levels** |
| **Mixed** | **Combination of aerobic and anaerobic activities** | **Fluctuates glucose levels** |

Figure 12.1 Aerobic exercise increases insulin sensitivity and, therefore, increases glucose uptake in the exercising muscles. Anaerobic exercise does not affect insulin sensitivity, and therefore, SBG remains high.

Exercise-induced hyperglycaemia can last for hours after an exercise session. This requires corrective insulin to be given, which in turn can increase the risk of late-onset hypoglycaemia, if the given insulin dose exceeds the required amount.

Many sporting activities typically involve both aerobic and anaerobic phases. Given the variability in glucose metabolism with both types of exercises, the glycaemic control of active type 1 diabetics can be challenging. In such situation, the continuous glucose monitoring (CGM) may be a useful addition to the management of blood glucose. CGM can also be used to study the effects of exercise on blood glucose and help in insulin adjustments and determining extra carbohydrate supplementation according to patient's activity.

> ### Three Steps for Diabetics Who Wish to Engage in Exercise
>
> 1. Pre-exercise medical checks
> 2. Advice on SBG monitoring and insulin dose adjustments
> 3. Customised prescription for all types of exercise (aerobic, non-aerobic, or both)

### Exercise with Insulin Pumps

The general principles of precaution and actions before, during, and after exercises in T1DM patients with insulin applies to those on continuous insulin infusion pumps (CIIP).

There are different pumps patients can select according to sporting needs. For example, a swimmer can obtain a waterproof CIIP. Insulin sensitivity increases during exercise/swimming. This sensitivity is affected to a large extent by the environmental temperature, intensity of exercise, and duration. Insulin dosage is basically reduced before exercise. If CIIP are temporarily removed before exercise, then a long-acting or intermediate insulin basal dose is given to cover for glycaemic control. Patients must ensure blood glucose is checked during and after exercises, and CIIP must be quickly reconnected.

---

- **Exercise improves insulin sensitivity in T2DM. Patients on insulin essentially require a reduction in insulin before engaging in exercise.**
- **Pre-exercise medical assessments are key.**
- **Before, during, and after exercise, SMBG allows patients to adjust insulin to prevent acute complications during exercise.**

---

# Driving with diabetes

How much diabetes affects driving is largely based on the type of diabetes, drug treatment, and presence of complications of diabetes. Safety at the wheels is very important due to hypoglycaemia in the driving diabetic.

Several steps must be taken to avoid this risk to oneself, those in the car, pedestrians and others using the roads.

### Informing Driving Authorities

All drivers are encouraged to inform their driving regulators of their diagnosis to seek appropriate advice regarding driving rules related to diabetes. In the United Kingdom, drivers are legally bounded to inform the Driving Vehicle Licensing Authority (DVLA) of their diagnosis, especially T2DM taking hypoglycaemic agents and T1DM on insulin therapy and those with complications of diabetes. DVLA provides advice and temporary license suspensions and reissues licenses depending on the state of diabetes control.

### Treatment with Oral Hypoglycaemic Agents (OHGA)

Certain OHGAs, such as the sulphonylureas and the glitinides, have hypoglycaemic effects. Diabetes UK recommends that precautions include: [12]

- Do not drive if your blood glucose is less than 4 mmol/l or your blood sugar has been under 4 mmol/l within the last forty-five minutes

- Keep your blood glucose above 5 mmol/l when driving
- Test your blood glucose levels within two hours of each journey
- Test your blood sugar every two hours whilst driving
- Keep a hypo treatment within reach for every drive

Group two (bus and lorry) licence holders at risk of hypos will need to have a record of blood tests on the memory of a blood glucose metre. This is so safety to drive can be assessed.

Keep hold of any blood glucose metres you have used in the last three months.

### Driving on Insulin

The risk of hypoglycaemia during driving is high. Therefore:

- Before driving, all drivers on insulin are advised to check their blood sugars every two hours until the end of the journey
- Should the driver develop symptoms of hypoglycaemia, the driver *must* pull aside, stop the engine, and take a fast-acting carbohydrate such as glucose tablets or sweets and some long-acting carbohydrates such as biscuits.
- Drivers should wait to drive for forty-five minutes after blood sugar level reaches ≥ 5 mmol.

Drivers who lose hypoglycaemic awareness will temporarily lose their license. Those who are initiated on insulin will also lose their license temporarily until they are used to insulin use and when they develop awareness of hypoglycaemic symptoms.

### Driving with Complications of Diabetes

Patients who have developed diabetes complications such as neuropathy and retinopathy will lose their license, as these complications affect the safety of their drive.

## Fasting with Diabetes

Many diabetic patients today decide to fast for religious beliefs and/or cultural purposes, whilst many others do so for various other reasons. It is, therefore, very important for the HCP to ensure appropriate medical advice and guidance are provided for patients before they embark on fasting.

Several caveats must be addressed.

### Informed Decision to Fast

If patients have the capacity (can take the advice, digest the information, weigh the risks of hypoglycaemia, and make the decision), then the appropriate information on complications of fasting, treatment modifications, and monitoring must be delivered. However, pregnant women and those with concomitant diseases—such as CAD, heart failure, liver failure, and previous hypo episodes—and unstable newly diagnosed T1DM and T2DM must be advised not to fast.

*Pre-fasting Assessment of Glycaemic Control and Other Comorbidities*

Assess patients' glycaemic control and other comorbidities in the pre-fasting review. Inform patients of complications and signs of complications during the review.

- Hypoglycaemia
- Hyperglycaemia
- Ketoacidosis
- Dehydration and thrombosis

*Appropriate timing in Breaking of Fasting*

Patients must be informed that breaking of the fast is necessary if sugar drops to 3.3 mmol/l or >16 mmol/l. Inform patients of the importance of frequent monitoring during the fasting.

*Appropriate Tailoring of Treatment during Fasting*

There are no guidelines on how to tailor treatment during fasting. Several regimens for insulin management have been looked at suggest different approaches:

- T1DM are advised not to fast, but if they proceed, the insulin regimen needs adjustment
- Those on premix insulin should seek advice on adjustments
- Those on basal insulin plus short-acting insulin need adjustments of both types of insulin dosages and frequency

## Travelling with Diabetes

Although there are no studies about travelling with diabetes that could provide accurate evidence-based recommendations for optimal management of diabetic patients travelling across different time zones, extensive clinical experiences by individuals and institutions provide general guidance on optimal management.

The papers by Chandran and Pinsker provide two classic examples of such experiences that contribute to the understanding of management of diabetics on insulin traversing different time zones. [13, 14]

The essential concepts from these papers are:

- Two insulin regimens were used (basal-bolus dose regimen and insulin pump).
- Types of insulin used in these regimens were long-acting first-generation analogues insulin (glargine/ detemir) or intermediate insulin NPH as basal insulin and short-acting insulin analogues lispro/aspart/glulisine as bolus insulin.
- Dosages and frequencies were not changed in patients travelling either north or south of the equator.
- Insulin dosages and frequencies were only changed in those travelling east or west over five or more time zones.
- Timing of the first basal dose was synchronised with the place of embarkation. Bolus doses were taken according to the number of meals and blood glucose levels during the flight.
- 'Travel Dose' – half dose of basal insulin taken at 12 hours at arrival time when travelling Westward and the second half basal dose taken 12 hours later.
- Travelling within a twelve-hour time difference with basal bolus dose of NPH does not require any adjustments.

These concepts are demonstrated in **Figures 12.2 and 12.3**

Let's consider, for example, the insulin adjustment for a person travelling eastward/westward across ten different time zones, from London to Papua New Guinea (PNG) and vice versa.

Firstly, travelling from PNG to London is westward and requires twenty-two hours of travel. PNG is nine hours ahead of London. Departure from Port Moresby will be at 2 p.m, PNG time (1 a.m. London time) heading to Singapore en route to London. Arrival in Singapore will be at 8 pm, PNG time (7 a.m. London time). There is a transit of two hours in Singapore. Departure from Singapore will be at 11 pm PNG time (10am London time) and arrival in London will be at 1 pm PNG time but 4 a.m. London time the next day.

Using the steps illustrated in **Figure 12.2**, a diabetic patient on a basal bolus insulin regimen of glargine 20 units and lispro insulin 15units with every meal

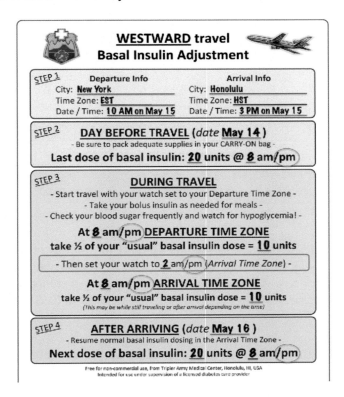

**Figure 12.2** Basal insulin calculation travelling Westward over > 5 time zones. Reproduced from Pinsker, J. E., Becker, E., Mahnke, C. B., Ching, M., Larson, N. S., & Roy, D. (2013, December 20). Extensive clinical experience: A simple guide to basal insulin adjustments for long-distance travel. *Journal of Diabetes and Metabolic Disorders*. BioMed Central Ltd. https://doi.org/10.1186/2251-6581-12-59

Starting from Step 2:
- Patient will take 20 units glargine at 8 a.m. as usual in PNG (on PNG time), 15 units lispro with every meal, and more/less if sugar is high/less inflight, with BG monitoring four to six times per day.
- Set time to London time zone

Step 3:
- Take half dose of 10 units glargine at 10pm London time (inflight). Patient will take next half dose of 10units 10am the next day, London time.
- Takes full dose of 20units glargine at 8am the next day

If the patient takes NPH 20 units bd, then he/she essentially maintains his/her dosages and frequencies but adjusts timing when arriving in London.

If the patient is travelling eastward from London to Port Moresby, steps in **Figure 12.3** can be used.

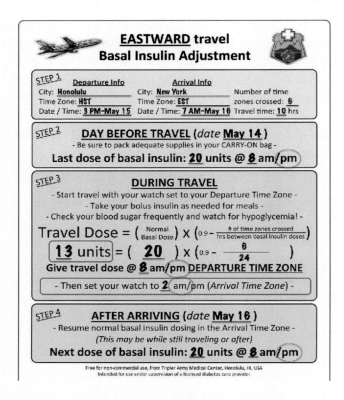

**Figure 12.3** Basal insulin calculation travelling Eastward. Reproduced from Pinsker, J. E., Becker, E., Mahnke, C. B., Ching, M., Larson, N. S., & Roy, D. (2013, December 20). Extensive clinical experience: A simple guide to basal insulin adjustments for long-distance travel. *Journal of Diabetes and Metabolic Disorders*. BioMed Central Ltd. https://doi.org/10.1186/2251-6581-12-59

Step 2:
- Patient will take 20units of glargine at 8am departure London time, checks glucose 3-4 times inflight
- Departs London at 4pm (London time) and sets time to arrival time zone
- Takes a travel dose of 9.6units of glargine at 6am (PNG time) on arrival in Singapore
- Takes another travel dose of 9.6 units glargine at 8am on arrival in PNG
- Takes a full 20units at 8am the next day in PNG

## Sick Day Rules

It is incumbent on the physician or the diabetic educator to provide sick day rules for all diabetic patients on diagnosis. These set of rules are guides for patients to follow when they are sick that will reduce their risks of developing complications and tell them when to call their doctors.

Patients must be educated and, preferably, given a written guide on what to do during times of sickness.

### Patients on OHGA

Patients on OHGA:

- May continue their meds, provided they maintain their carbohydrate intake (either solid or liquid) and blood glucose is monitored every four hours
- Must seek medical advice if blood glucose is >13 mmol/l
- Should stop metformin when dehydrated and may need to be admitted to hospital

## Patients on Insulin

Insulin should not be stopped as patients are at risk of hyperglycaemia during illness. In fact, insulin requirement increases during illness, and patients must be educated on when and how to increase insulin dosages.

In the absence of sick day rules, 'a rule of thumb':

- For BG <13 mmol/l, continue current dose of insulin
- For BG between 13 and 22 mmol/l, increase dose by 2 units per injection
- For BG >22 mmol/l increase dose by 4 units per injection, even if patient is not able to eat
- Reduce dose to normal if BG normalises

## Scheduled Blood Glucose (BG) and Ketone Testing

Regular and constant BG and ketone monitoring should be continued until BG <13 mml/l, patient is eating normally, and urine is negative for ketones.

Patients should test for ketonuria one to two times per day or more than that if ketones are present.

## Hydration

All diabetic patients must be advised on drinking lots of sugar-free fluids / water to keep hydrated during acute illness. Nausea and vomiting can be treated with antiemetics.

## Seeking Medical Advice

Patients must be informed and advised to seek medical advice when they:

- Are unable to eat or drink
- Have persistent diarrhoea or vomiting
- Have BG >25 mmol/l, even though they have increased insulin
- Have hypoglycaemia
- Have persistent ketones in urine
- Are confused or drowsy or when other concerns are present

---

### Sick Day Rules:

- Maintain adequate hydration
- Check BG regularly
- Maintain carbohydrate intake
- Increase insulin doses
- Seek medical advice when appropriate

---

## Key Messages:

- **Pregnancy screening and optimisation of glycaemic control prior to pregnancy will reduce pregnancy-related diabetes complications.**
- **Optimal partum and postpartum glycaemic management is critical for patients' successful outcomes.**

- **Patients who drink alcohol must be advised on post-drinking hypoglycaemia and how to prevent it.**
- **Newly diagnosed diabetes patients on OHGA or insulin must inform their driving authorities and cease driving until being cleared to drive.**
- **Treatment experienced patients must take certain precautions to avoid hypoglycaemia during driving.**
- **Travelling different time zones with diabetes requires adjustments of insulin dosages and timing.**
- **Insulin must be continued and increase during sick days, with regular monitoring. Patients must be informed when to present to hospital.**

## References

1  Holmes, V. A., Young, I. S., Patterson, C. C.,et.al., & Diabetes and Pre-eclampsia Intervention Trial Study Group (2011). Optimal glycemic control, pre-eclampsia, and gestational hypertension in women with type 1 diabetes in the diabetes and pre-eclampsia intervention trial. *Diabetes care*, *34*(8), 1683–1688. https://doi.org/10.2337/dc11-0244

2  ACOG Practice Bulletin No. 190: Gestational Diabetes Mellitus. (2018). *Obstetrics and gynecology*, *131*(2), e49–e64. https://doi.org/10.1097/AOG.0000000000002501

3  Crowther, C. A., Hiller, J. E., Moss, J. R., McPhee, A. J., Jeffries, W. S., Robinson, J. S., & Australian Carbohydrate Intolerance Study in Pregnant Women (ACHOIS) Trial Group (2005). Effect of treatment of gestational diabetes mellitus on pregnancy outcomes. *The New England journal of medicine*, *352*(24), 2477–2486. https://doi.org/10.1056/NEJMoa042973

4  Hartling, L., Dryden, D. M., Guthrie, A., Muise, M., Vandermeer, B., & Donovan, L. (2013). Benefits and harms of treating gestational diabetes mellitus: a systematic review and meta-analysis for the U.S. Preventive Services Task Force and the National Institutes of Health Office of Medical Applications of Research. *Annals of internal medicine*, *159*(2), 123–129. https://doi.org/10.7326/0003-4819-159-2-201307160-00661

5  Gilbert, C., Valois, M., & Koren, G. (2006). Pregnancy outcome after first-trimester exposure to metformin: a meta-analysis. *Fertility and sterility*, *86*(3), 658–663. https://doi.org/10.1016/j.fertnstert.2006.02.098

6  Hebert, M. F., Ma, X., Naraharisetti, S. B., Krudys, et.al., & Obstetric-Fetal Pharmacology Research Unit Network (2009). Are we optimizing gestational diabetes treatment with glyburide? The pharmacologic basis for better clinical practice. *Clinical pharmacology and therapeutics*, *85*(6), 607–614. https://doi.org/10.1038/clpt.2009.5

7  Carlsson, S., Hammar, N., & Grill, V. (2005). Alcohol consumption and type 2 diabetes Meta-analysis of epidemiological studies indicates a U-shaped relationship. *Diabetologia*, *48*(6), 1051–1054. https://doi.org/10.1007/s00125-005-1768-5

8  Dalal Alromaihi, Judith Zielke, Arti Bhan; Challenges of Type 2 Diabetes in Patients With Alcohol Dependence. *Clin Diabetes* 1 July 2012; 30 (3): 120–122. https://doi.org/10.2337/diaclin.30.3.120

9  Alcohol-use disorders: diagnosis, assessment and management of harmful drinking (high-risk drinking) and alcohol dependence. Clinical guideline [CG115]. https://www.nice.org.uk/guideline/cg115/chapter/key-priorities-for-implementation

10  W. Guyton Hornsby, Robert D. Chetlin; Management of Competitive Athletes With Diabetes. *Diabetes Spectr* 1 April 2005; 18 (2): 102–107. https://doi.org/10.2337/diaspect.18.2.102

11  Colberg, S. R., Sigal, R. J., Fernhall, B., Regensteiner, J. G., Blissmer, B. J., Rubin, R. R., Chasan-Taber, L., Albright, A. L., Braun, B., American College of Sports Medicine, & American Diabetes Association (2010). Exercise and type 2 diabetes: the American College of Sports Medicine and the American Diabetes Association: joint position statement. *Diabetes care*, *33*(12), e147–e167. https://doi.org/10.2337/dc10-9990

12  Diabetes UK.Driving with Diabetes. https://www.diabetes.co.uk/driving-with-diabetes.html

13  Manju Chandran, Steven V. Edelman; Have Insulin, Will Fly: Diabetes Management During Air Travel and Time Zone Adjustment Strategies. *Clin Diabetes* 1 April 2003; 21 (2): 82–85. https://doi.org/10.2337/diaclin.21.2.82

14  Pinsker, J. E., Becker, E., Mahnke, C. B., Ching, M., Larson, N. S., & Roy, D. (2013). Extensive clinical experience: a simple guide to basal insulin adjustments for long-distance travel. *Journal of diabetes and metabolic disorders*, *12*(1), 59. https://doi.org/10.1186/2251-6581-12-59

# Index

Printed in the United States
by Baker & Taylor Publisher Services